MODERN EPIDEMICS

MODERN EPIDEMICS

From the Spanish Flu to COVID-19

Salvador Macip

Translated from Catalan by Julie Wark

polity

LLLL institut
ramon llull

This book has been supported by the Institut Ramon Llull

Polity Press
65 Bridge Street
Cambridge CB2 1UR, UK

Polity Press
101 Station Landing
Suite 300
Medford, MA 02155, USA

ISBN-13: 978-1-5095-4656-5 - hardback
ISBN-13: 978-1-5095-4657-2 - paperback

A catalogue record for this book is available from the British Library.

Typeset in 10.75pt on 14pt Janson by
Servis Filmsetting Limited, Stockport, Cheshire
Printed and bound in Great Britain by TJ Books Ltd, Padstow, Cornwall

The publisher has used its best endeavours to ensure that the URLs for external websites referred to in this book are correct and active at the time of going to press. However, the publisher has no responsibility for the websites and can make no guarantee that a site will remain live or that the content is or will remain appropriate.

For further information on Polity, visit our website: politybooks.com

For my mother:

Thank you for all these years of unconditional support

The smallest unit of life – a single bacterial cell – is a monument of pattern and process unrivalled in the universe as we know it.

Lynn Margulis and Dorion Sagan, *Microcosmos:
Four Billion Years of Microbial Evolution* (University of
California Press, 1986)

But there is something terrifying about the fact that nothing can stop the implacable evolution of these viruses as they test, through mindless mutation, ever more strategies to facilitate their survival, a survival that just may represent disease and death for us humans.

C. J. Peters and Mark Olshaker, *Virus Hunter:
Thirty Years of Battling Hot Viruses around the World*
(Anchor Books, 1997)

Contents

Acknowledgements

My thanks to colleagues who guided my first steps in the fascinating world of studying microorganisms: Dr Luca Gusella, Dr Arantxa Horga, Dr Adolfo García-Sastre and Dr Luis Martínez-Sobrido. And more thanks for the deliberations and conversations that have ended up appearing in this book. A thousand thanks to Dr Jordi Gómez i Prat, Dr Marta Giralt, Dr Joan Fontdevila and Dr Ana Fernández Sesma for their help, their selfless supervision, and for letting me interview them. Another thousand to C. J. Peters, L. Margulis, D. Sagan, D. H. Crawford, D. Grady, G. Kolata and M. Siegel for their books on the subject, which have been my references.

My gratitude to Gonzalo Pontón for his contribution in giving shape to this project, to Pau Centellas and Carlota Torrents for their part in bringing into being what finally ended up as a book, to Emili Rosales and Ramón Perelló for enabling the project grow, to Isabel Martí and Josep Maria Espinàs for their guidance in polishing it, and to John Thompson and Elise Heslinga for helping me turn it into a much better book.

As always, my thanks to Yolanda, Pol, Antoni-Jordi, Josefina and Ana for being at my side, for helping me in difficult moments, and for being unsparing with their criticism.

Introduction

An ever-present danger

In spring 2009, there was an outbreak in Mexico of an influenza pandemic that spread unstoppably around the world in just a few weeks. Many people were taken by surprise as they hadn't imagined that, with all the advances in medicine today, we could still feel so helpless when faced with such a common virus. Yet, scientists had been predicting it for quite some time. When the first edition of this book was published, over a decade ago, by which time that pandemic had started to abate, I was interviewed by some newspapers and repeated the same thing several times: it was indisputable that there would be another pandemic in a few years' time, and we had better prepare in case the virus that would be circulating then turned out to be more aggressive than A(H1N1), the so-called 'swine flu' virus, which was creating so many problems. Such long-term prophecies are easy to make because, if you are wrong, no one remembers, so you don't get taken to task about it afterwards. But, in this case, it wasn't prediction but certainty. All the experts I had spoken to or read while writing this book agreed that it was inevitable. Everyone who had sufficiently studied the matter came to the same conclusion: it wasn't a matter of waiting to see *if* it would happen but *when* it would happen.

When I said this, people looked at me not so much with fear as with an amused or incredulous expression. Another alarmist, they must have thought. In the Epilogue of this book, I explain how the publishers of the first version were also surprised when I anticipated the 2009 pandemic some months before it happened. They had an excuse, because they hadn't experienced an infectious disease of such dimensions, but the attitude should have changed after the A(H1N1) flu, which could be regarded as the first pandemic of the modern era, the first to have attacked a globalized, frontierless world. This should have warned us of what can happen when, faced with the appearance of an unknown virus against which we have no defences, we are obliged to act swiftly in order to avert a possible tragedy. But, even so, the outbreak of COVID-19, the disease caused by the new virus called SARS-CoV-2, caught us unawares.

The responses to this second great twenty-first century world health crisis (in terms of viruses) are very similar to those of the first one, namely confusion, panic and uncertainty. Once again, mismanaged information has sown distrust among the public. Perhaps there is one slight improvement in that many countries have responded faster and have shared important data more efficiently. Despite the doubts and unnecessary delays of the early weeks, protective measures are now being more firmly applied. Yet, there are many issues still to be resolved if we want to be better prepared for future pandemics.

Fortunately, SARS-CoV-2 isn't the 'supervirus' that I talk about later in these pages, but it does raise more logistical problems than any of the flu viruses we've seen recently. Although we are still not well enough informed about it, we do know that it spreads very fast (partly because those affected are contagious for a long period without symptoms), and that it has a relatively low mortality rate of probably somewhere near 1 per cent. To give some perspective, this is ten times higher than the 0.1 per cent for seasonal flu but much lower than the 50–80 per cent for Ebola. If we add up these factors, as well as the many uncertainties, there are more than enough reasons to be cautious and to act as fast as possible. It's true that the symptoms it presents are relatively mild in most cases, but in some, especially for certain groups of the population (for example, elderly people and those with serious illnesses), it can be fatal. This, together with the great ease of contagion, can create very serious problems of global health, which is why it is essential to prevent its spread as soon as possible.

However, although COVID-19 is taking up so much media space, it isn't the only infectious disease we should be worried about. In terms of health impact, the four big epidemics and pandemics are still influenza, AIDS, malaria and tuberculosis. It's true that we've recently had the biggest Ebola outbreak in history, but it's still a disease that is restricted to certain areas of the globe. At the same time, we've seen how the coronavirus family has gained prominence, and how these microbes are capable of creating worldwide alerts. The first serious illness caused by these viruses was SARS which, though it was seen as a possible long-term risk at the beginning of the century, appears to be fairly well under control for the moment. After SARS, in 2012 there was MERS (Middle East Respiratory Syndrome), but this, too, remained quite localized. It wasn't until the appearance of the third great coronavirus, SARS-CoV-2, that all the alarms went off.

So, are the coronaviruses the latest danger for humanity? Would they deserve a chapter alongside the other four major infectious diseases? Right now, it's hard to know. Coronaviruses usually come from bats, which act as reservoirs, the places where the viruses survive and reproduce. And it's highly probable that other strains will end up jumping to humans in areas where there's more contact with animals (and China is one of the main loci of the problem because of its traditions and lax regulation of public markets where wild animals are sold). But we will need to wait and see whether or not this ends up becoming a major health problem in the coming decades.

As for COVID-19, its impact will depend on how quickly an effective vaccine is found, produced and administered, and on the virus's ability to keep changing. It seems clear that it's a big enough threat to be taken seriously, and that it's going to cause major problems for quite some time. But, the most likely thing is that we will end up getting the better of it, if all goes well. It's possible that, afterwards, there will still be outbreaks but, in normal circumstances – once a good part of the population has a certain immunity after coming into contact with the virus, and when we have the appropriate complementary tools (vaccine, antivirals, and so on) – it would never cause another pandemic like that of 2020. Nevertheless, this doesn't mean that we can lower our guard. I must insist that there will be more pandemics, and the danger that one of them will be caused by an even more aggressive virus is always going to be present.

Let's do our homework

Meanwhile, what can we do? Prepare ourselves for the future. It's easy to forget the latent problem of pandemics when we've just overcome one and, in statistical terms, it's not very likely that the next one will appear any time soon. But governments have the obligation to plan rapid response measures and, even more important, to instruct the population. Unless people – all the people – participate, we won't be able to confront infections with any guarantee of success. We've already seen this twice in the twenty-first century: when there's a crisis at the global level, it's necessary to count on everyone to root out the problem. The conclusions we can draw in 2020 are the same as those reached in 2009. Most importantly: when a new virus appears, rapid, coordinated action is necessary until we understand the extent of the symptoms it's causing, even if they seem mild at first. And we can only achieve this if we all understand how an infectious disease works and what the real power of microbes is.

Though it may seem excessive, isolating infected populations, encouraging hygiene and avoiding large gatherings of people are highly effective strategies in these situations, especially when it comes to making sure that the disease doesn't cause its own particular kind of collapse of a country's health system, which would end up with many collateral victims. This is crucial in the early phases of an epidemic. But it's also necessary to improve public management of the crisis, which is invariably one of the weak points. And there will always be someone who believes the whole thing is a plot or an exaggeration, but we must manage to ensure that this position remains marginal, and that people listen to those who know what they are talking about. Hence, there needs to be a sound, well-coordinated communication strategy and, if possible, one with a single, reliable source of information (maybe the WHO, or maybe a new body) backed by all the authorities and the media and making the details widely available. And all of us also need to make an effort to learn a bit more about microbes.

SARS and MERS have been warnings of the danger that a microbe from this family could represent in the right conditions, and scientists spoke out loud and clear to announce it. Many people thought they were exaggerating because neither of the two epidemics turned out to be as serious as originally predicted. Now, with millions affected by COVID-19, from Asia to America and everywhere in-between, the fear of being vulnerable to the microbes around us has become generalized. Which position is more correct? Shrugging it off to the point of ignoring the experts' warnings, or panicking about going outside and breathing air that's full of invisible killers? The best idea, of course, is to find a middle course.

However, in order to make these kinds of decisions, we need clear information about the present risks of suffering from a serious infection and what we can do to prevent it. It isn't always easy to obtain this because we are constantly finding clashing opinions in the media, ranging from those announcing an apocalypse to others who believe there is nothing to worry about. Who is right? We must respect viruses and bacteria and understand that we can't always defeat them, and now, well into the twenty-first century, we also need to know the extent to which it's possible that a pandemic can cause millions of deaths, as has happened several times throughout history.

A tool for understanding the present and preparing for the future

This is where we scientists can help a little. Popular science books like this can make a humble contribution to general knowledge and, in doing so, gradually ensure that microbes cease to be the great unknowns we only talk about when it's already too late. Here, you will find some tools offering a better understanding of how infections work and what resources we have for stopping them. This information could be useful in the future, but it has special relevance now when COVID-19 has caused such an upheaval to our way of life. That is the reasoning behind publication of this updated, expanded edition, which includes everything we know so far about coronaviruses.

In the following pages, I've tried to fill in the gaps in general knowledge about microbes and to provide readers with a direct account of, and basic data about, such common but, in fact, little understood diseases like flu and AIDS, which are caused by the most important microbes. On some fronts of our struggle against infections, we remain in a tactical draw, with no guarantees that the situation will continue like this indefinitely. On others, we are clearly losing the game. And according to some experts, the situation can get worse at any time and we won't be able to do anything to prevent it. We shouldn't even count on our few victories because all the ground we've gained could be lost overnight if we are not careful.

Few fields arouse as much fear and incomprehension as microbiology, the study of invisible organisms that are as likely to help us to survive as to wipe us off the face of the Earth. In recent years, we've not only seen the spectre of influenza making front-page news; we've also learned to live with AIDS – the most significant pandemic our species has suffered for centuries – and to such an extent that many people have lost respect for it. We've heard news of the advance of a type of tuberculosis that can't be cured with any drug, but we think that this is a problem that will never affect us. Thanks to irresponsible media campaigns, we've become so scared of vaccines that child health has regressed by several decades. We've discovered that a small amount of white powder inside an envelope can keep a whole country terrified for months. We've feared that the next war could be fought by throwing deadly bacteria at civilian populations. We've seen how the military considered that a disease we believed was eradicated could be more effective than an atomic bomb. And lurking behind all this are always the same culprits: microbes.

We must realize that viruses and bacteria haven't only shaped the history of humanity, they are also responsible for millions of deaths, although they are not always front-page news. We need to know the subject well enough not to be flummoxed by the inflated reports we find in the media but, at the same time, to know when we have to act quickly. We must be aware of the strategies we have within our reach for combating microorganisms and the extent to which they can protect us. And, above all, we need to put an end to a series of myths and false beliefs that are hindering advances in the area of health. My aim as an educator is to remedy some of these shortcomings.

The book is divided into two parts, which are independent and can be read in the order the reader prefers. In the first, more general part, I will give an account of what microorganisms are and describe some of the historic pandemics that have seriously threatened our survival. The second part focuses on the main infectious diseases we haven't yet managed to control; namely, what we can rightly call the four great modern plagues: influenza, AIDS, tuberculosis and malaria. They are important because of the number of people they affect around the world, their serious economic and social impact, their aggressiveness and, in some cases, the scant means we still have for fighting them. Some have already spread all over the planet. Others are circumscribed to certain areas, but that doesn't mean they don't cause large numbers of casualties. I will assess how far we are from defeating them and the risks of seeing them turning into tragedies beyond our control. I will also discuss, in particular, the gravity of the present pandemic and how it's expected to evolve.

In this book, I want to raise several questions that I believe are necessary. Does our future depend on microorganisms? Why do antibiotics stop being effective? How much longer will they serve us? Will an AIDS vaccine ever be found? Or a cure? Why are we so afraid of influenza coming from animals, like bird or swine flu? Could a flu epidemic today wipe out half the world's population? Do we have the means to stop dangerous infections before they spread? Should we fear an attack with biological weapons? Are we immune to infectious diseases that have been eradicated? What can we do to avoid being infected? Can vaccines cause autism? We will now move on to delve into the fascinating world of viruses and bacteria in order to find the answers.

I don't think anyone would doubt today that infectious diseases are a global problem. They start in one corner of the planet, but our lifestyle helps them to spread like wildfire. Pandemics are still frequent, and we must learn from every episode so we can do better next time. These are problems we can't ignore. I hope this book will help readers to see what it means to share the planet with all these invisible enemies and that, at the end of the day, we will be able to find together that much-needed point between alarm and caution which will allow us to survive as a species for many more millennia.

Part I

Sharing the World with Microorganisms

1

Travel Companions

We humans have managed to escape from our predators. In the security of urban settings, we don't have to worry about being devoured by lions, tigers or other carnivores that are stronger and faster than we are. As a result, we've successfully occupied all the ecosystems and multiply like no other animal has ever done before. We therefore tend to think we are invulnerable, at least when it comes to competing with other inhabitants of the Earth for our everyday survival.

This idea couldn't be more wrong. We are immersed in a constant struggle against an adversary so powerful it can eliminate the human race in a matter of months. Indeed, it's been on the point of doing so more than once. I refer to microorganisms, our invisible enemies, the millions of microscopic beings sharing our habitat, the bacteria, viruses and many other minuscule life forms with which we have a very special love–hate relationship. Thanks to them, we're alive. Because of them, some 14 million people die every year. Why are we still vulnerable to such infinitesimal organisms? This chapter will introduce the main kinds of microbes and describe how they interact with humans.

They were here first

Microbes are the oldest inhabitants of this planet. They've been around for between 3,000 and 4,000 million years, but humans didn't discover them until a little more than a century ago when science was sufficiently advanced to let us see them close up with the aid of a microscope. During the first 2,000 million years, microbes, and specifically bacteria, had the Earth to themselves. They were the first to appear and will doubtless be the last to leave because they are not only the most diverse form of life but are also the one that most easily adapts to any conditions. If a catastrophe wiped out most life on Earth, they would probably be the only survivors.

There are more than a million kinds of microorganisms, most of them inoffensive. The main ones are bacteria and viruses, but to these must be added certain fungi, algae and amoebas. In both number and weight, microorganisms are predominant among living beings. If we could put all the microbes on one side of the scale and all the animals on the other, the microbes would weigh twenty-five times more. The fastest growing microbes duplicate every thirteen minutes, and the slowest every fourteen days. At this rate, if a single bacterium had all the possible nutrients and the right conditions, it could generate a colony that would weigh as much as the whole Earth in three days.

We shouldn't forget that it's thanks to microbes that this planet is habitable. Some 2,700 million years ago, there appeared a certain kind of bacterium that was able to use

Space: the last frontier

Bacteria could also survive in outer space. Some very tiny species have been found (among them *Herminiimonas glaciei*, which was discovered in 2009). They can endure for more than 120,000 years under layers of ice three kilometres thick, practically without oxygen and nutrients. These conditions are very similar to those that might be found outside our planet.

sunlight to transform water and CO_2 into energy. A secondary effect of this process, which is called *photosynthesis*, is generation of oxygen. Like toxic exhaust fumes given off by a car engine, the oxygen kept accumulating in huge quantities and 'contaminating' the Earth's atmosphere. This inadvertent pollution ended up being providential for us as it permitted the appearance of a new class of beings – humans among them – that needed oxygen for their basic functions. To this very day, bacteria are important for keeping the planet in balance. Without them, life on Earth would be wiped out.

We should be grateful for other things, too. Bacteria are also our ancestors. As I said, life on Earth was at first limited to minuscule single cell organisms. They gradually began to come together in groups of cells that, acting in concert, went on to specialize in different functions, now in the form of what are known as *multicellular* organisms. This is the path that led to the fabulous biological diversity we have today. As proof of our humble origins, there are still structures in human cells that come directly from those original bacteria. And they are essential for human life.

Peaceful passengers

We shouldn't necessarily see microorganisms as a threat. On the contrary, coexistence with many of them is highly beneficial for humans and determines proper functioning of the organism. The human body, one of the most complex multicellular organisms in existence, consists of approximately 100 billion cells. But this needs to be clarified: I mean 100 billion *human* cells. If we are to be exact, we also need to count all the microorganisms that inhabit us. Initially, it was calculated that they might be ten times more numerous than our own cells, but more recent data suggest that a closer estimate would be one microbe for each human cell. In any case, we can venture that the human body is colonized by millions of microorganisms, of some 400 different species, which normally don't cause any illness. Put together they would weigh a kilogram. These data are mind-boggling, enough to make us wonder what a human being really is. A mixture of highly specialized cells and microbes that live in harmony? From this standpoint, we are perhaps nothing more than a walking ecosystem in which a series of microorganisms peaceably survive.

The microbes that are always with us are not only freeloaders but 'stowaways' that are very important for our metabolism. Humans, like all other animals, depend on them to survive. From them, we obtain vitamins, nutrients and protection against infections caused by their more toxic kin. Cows, for example, couldn't ingest grass without the help of the bacteria they have in their digestive tract, and neither could termites benefit from the cellulose in wood. There are plants we use as food, peas and beans for example, that need bacteria in order to fix the essential nitrogen from the sun.

Further proof of their importance is that it is thought that,

Nomenclature

By convention, microorganisms, like all other living beings, are designated by using a first name (with the first letter capitalized) and a second name, both in Latin. The first is the genus name and the second the species name. The genus name can be abbreviated to the initial alone, and both tend to be italicized. Example: *Mycobacterium tuberculosis* (or *M. tuberculosis*) is a species of bacteria of the genus of microbacteria that causes tuberculosis.

when giving birth, mothers pass on to their children the 'good' bacteria that will settle in their digestive systems and protect them in the future. Hence, there are studies exploring what happens to babies born by caesarean, because these children haven't had to pass through the vaginal canal that would equip them with their first microorganisms. It's not yet sure what effect this might have on their future health.

In the domain of health, more and more importance is being given to what's known as the *microbiota*, or the set of all the microorganisms each person carries inside (and on the surface). It's believed that, depending on which microbes inhabit this microbiota, we can be more or less prone to certain illnesses or conditions.

One example of this would be that the type of bacteria found in intestines could determine whether we gain weight or not, as was first suggested in a study from 2006. After isolating intestinal bacteria from mice of normal weight and from others that were obese, scientists found that bacteria from the latter contributed towards weight gain in the former, even when they continued with the same diet. Humans have between 500 and 1,000 different species of bacteria in the digestive tract and it might well be that these also have an influence on a person's susceptibility to gaining weight. More recent studies support this theory. For example, in 2009 it was found that obese women have a high presence in their saliva of bacteria called *Selenomonas noxia*. By contrast, thin women show a very different set of bacteria.

Secondary effects

It's been known for some time now that antibiotics can disrupt the balance of 'good' bacteria. Medicines eliminate infections but are unable to distinguish between aggressive and innocuous microbes. Depending on the treatment, even weeks can go by in some cases before the bacterial composition of the intestine, for example, completely recovers. This can then give rise to diarrhoea or new infections caused by other harmful bacteria, especially in people already weakened by illness.

This shows that it is not only our intestines that are full of microorganisms. Our mouths, too, normally have between six and thirty different types of bacteria. And skin is another organ that is home to thousands more. It was once believed that most of them were of the genus *Staphylococcus*, because when samples taken from human skin were cultivated in the laboratory, they were the most visible. But this doesn't mean that there aren't many more. There are others that don't divide so quickly. Indeed, with the new tools of genetic analysis, it's been possible to see that the set of denizens of human skin is much more complex than was previously thought, with up to 1,000 different species, which is to say, a number that's comparable with that for the intestines. The skin behind the ear is the zone with the least diversity of bacteria, with only fifteen kinds, while the forearm has as many as forty-four. This varying distribution might explain why-some skin diseases appear in certain zones and not in others. As in the intestines, bacteria on the skin have important functions, so, for example, oilier zones have some bacteria that produce a moisturizing substance to stop the skin from cracking.

In recent years, several studies have set about the task of identifying all the microorganisms that are to be found in different organs, generally using modern techniques to read their genes in order to relate them to obesity or illness. These studies give us a general idea of the microbes we carry around with us, although each person's flora is, in fact, unique. Almost like our DNA. It depends more on the zone in which we live than on our genes, and personal habits have a considerable influence as well. An article published in January 2009 demonstrated that sets of intestinal bacteria vary even between twins. Nevertheless, the members of a family living under the same roof have similar flora. The article also indicated that obesity reduces the diversity of flora, as well as altering the genes and metabolism of microorganisms. It's speculated that this might have consequences for our health, but we still aren't sure what they might be.

This knowledge we are acquiring about the microbes that coexist with us has led to questions about whether they can be used for therapeutic purposes. There are now studies looking into ways of changing the composition of a person's microbiota as a way of curing illnesses and even regulating the metabolism with the aim of weight loss. The easiest way is to take microbes from a healthy person's faeces and transfer them to the patient. Informally known as a stool transplant, this isn't such a simple process as it may appear, because it requires, first of all, filtering out the bad microbes and other contaminants.

It's still not known whether this procedure might have any

real benefit, but what is undeniable is that the microbiota plays an important role in our health, both positively and negatively. This could be more far-reaching than initially imagined. Some studies have even shown that the microbes inhabiting our intestines could affect the brain and somehow influence behaviour.

The dark side

It's well known that not all microbes are as beneficial as the ones I've just described. A group called *pathogens*, amounting to only 1,415 of all those that exist, have been found to cause infectious diseases in humans. Although they are clearly a minority, their impact on society has been, and is, immense.

Infections occur when one of these pathogens manages to enter our organism and overcome its defence systems. Problems arise when the microbe starts drawing on the resources of the organisms it has invaded to multiply nonstop. If this isn't checked fast enough, it will end up interfering with the normal functioning of the body, presenting the symptoms characteristic of each infection, depending on the organs the invader prefers. Some of these symptoms are shared by many infectious diseases, for example, fever, shivers or feeling unwell in general.

It's commonly believed that, thanks to the discovery of antibiotics, pathogenic microbes have ceased to be the terrible threat they were until just a few decades ago. To some extent, this is true. Nevertheless, we are a long way from being able to feel relaxed about this. On the one hand, bacteria that are resistant to the most commonly used antibiotics are constantly appearing. On the other, some serious illnesses still exist for which there are no vaccines or treatment.

And there are still others that have both but, even so, we can't stop them. Moreover, it should be recalled that antibiotics are only useful against bacteria, but they don't work with viruses. It's true that we have antivirals to fight these microbes, but they aren't so effective, and we still haven't produced such a wide range either. This, then, is a never-ending struggle.

A bit of terminology

With regard to infections, there's a series of terms that are frequently used to define their reach. For example, an *outbreak* is an infection localized among a relatively small group of people, for example, a family, a school or even a village. A typical case would be food poisoning, which tends to affect only those who have eaten food containing pathogenic microbes.

The next level is an *epidemic*, which is defined rather arbitrarily as an accumulation of infected people that's bigger than 'normal'. For example, if a disease is very rare, a mere handful of cases could be regarded as an epidemic. When an epidemic has spread through more than a continent or even the whole planet, we call it a *pandemic*. Technically speaking, the WHO officially declares a pandemic only when a disease goes beyond six phases, ranging from detection of the microbe in animals (phase 1) through to the continuing presence of the disease in more than one of the regions defined by the organization (phase 6).

An infectious disease that's constantly present in a region without any significant fall or rise in the number of cases is said to be *endemic*. For example, malaria is endemic to many parts of Africa. Whether or not an outbreak turns into an epidemic, a pandemic or becomes endemic depends on many factors, among them the speed at which it spreads and the virulence of the disease it causes.

Which disease spreads fastest?

It has been estimated that the 1918 flu pandemic had an R0 of around 4 (meaning that each affected person infected four more). Seasonal flu (the annual one) normally has an R0 of between 1.3 and 3. The A(H1N1) flu pandemic of spring 2009 had an R0 of only 1.4, while that for measles is 15, which means that it's a much more contagious disease than the others. The R0 for smallpox was between 5 and 10, and for AIDS it's between 10 and 12. That for COVID-19 is still being calculated, but it could be close to 2 at the very most.

An infection's ability to spread is defined by a variable called *R0*, which is to say the number of new infections that, on average, each person with the disease can cause or, in other words, how many more people can catch the disease from each already infected person (see box). It's also important to know the amount of time over which a person can infect others. With most infectious diseases there's a period of incubation when, although the symptoms haven't yet appeared, the microbe can often be transmitted. The longer the period, the greater the risk of the outbreak spreading because the infected person normally doesn't know and appropriate measures to avoid contagion aren't taken. One known example of this is COVID-19, which, going unnoticed in the early (between ten and fifteen) days, can be contagious. The extreme case is AIDS, which may not show any signs for years. In some cases, infected people will never develop the disease but can, nevertheless, pass it on to others. They're called *carriers*.

Typhoid Mary

Mary Mallon (1869–1938) has gone down in history as 'Typhoid Mary', the first person to be identified in the United States as a carrier of typhoid fever (a disease caused by the bacteria *Salmonella*, which is transmitted through contaminated food or drink) without ever being ill herself. Mary was a kind of epidemic on two legs. She infected fifty-three people in her lifetime but always denied that she was to blame. Moreover, she never wanted to leave her job as a cook, despite the very high chances that she would infect people through the food she prepared. When she was banned from cooking, she even changed her name so she could keep doing her job and thus continue to infect and kill her clients.

Mary, who worked in New York, was finally forced to go into quarantine. When she died (of pneumonia) she was still in isolation. It's believed that she could have been born with the infection, as her mother had the disease when she was pregnant.

The other important factor when defining the aggressiveness of an outbreak is the severity of the symptoms it causes. These can range from a slight fever and feeling out of sorts (as with the common cold) to death. It's said that the *virulence* of the infection is determined by the intensity of the effects it has in people. An infection that spreads quickly (one with a high R0) usually has low virulence, but, even so, it can still constitute a major health problem, as we've seen with COVID-19. Then again, if a disease kills a high percentage of infected people, the ease of contagion tends to be much lower, so it's unlikely to cause a pandemic (as it will remain localized). A typical example of this would be Ebola, which has very high lethality, but it rarely goes beyond an outbreak or, at most, an epidemic. A combination of easy transmission and high virulence is what is most dangerous. Fortunately, this combination is highly improbable.

Animals are sometimes part of infectious cycles in which they become *reservoirs* – that is to say, a place where microbes can accumulate and from which they can infect humans in future. Very often, the animals that act as reservoirs aren't affected by the presence of the microbes and show no symptoms of disease either. The existence of reservoirs makes it very difficult to eliminate microbes completely. Examples include pigs and birds (common reservoirs of influenza viruses), and mosquitoes (reservoirs of malaria). Many of the major recent pandemics come from viruses that have jumped to humans from their reservoir animals, for example monkeys in the case of AIDS and, probably, bats in that of COVID-19.

Bacteria

To conclude this initial chapter, I will give a brief account of the three most important kinds of microorganisms from the medical point of view: bacteria, viruses and fungi.

Bacteria are microbes consisting of a single cell. After the sixteenth century, there were theories postulating that diseases were transmitted by a kind of 'seed' that went from one person to another but, without the necessary instruments, it was impossible to confirm this idea. It wasn't until the seventeenth century, when the Dutchman Antonie van Leeuwenhoek invented the microscope, that it was possible to discover these 'germs', as they were originally called. In one of his first observations, he described something like abundant 'very little animalcules', which were everywhere. He named them *animalculae* and proposed that they were responsible for infections. It was only possible to demonstrate this in the nineteenth century and, in 1838, Leeuwenhoek's *animalculae* were officially named bacteria.

There are many classes of bacteria and they can have very different forms. The most typical are round and they're called *cocci*, while the elongated ones are known as *bacilli*. They are found everywhere, and in abundance. For example, there are 40 million bacteria in every gram of earth, and 1 million for each millilitre of water. If we counted all the bacteria on the planet, we would get a figure with thirty zeros. It's therefore believed that most of the types that exist haven't yet been discovered or identified.

As I said in the beginning, bacteria participate in many important processes in our ecosystems, for example recycling nutrients through nitrogen fixation and putrefaction. They are also necessary for fermentation: without the work of bacteria, there would be no cheese, wine, vinegar or yoghurt. Scientific advances have made it possible for us to carry out research with them in laboratories, and new bioengineering techniques allow us to use them to produce insulin and antibodies.

Bacteria multiply by means of a process called *binary fission*, during which a bacterium divides into two identical parts. The genetic information of a bacterium is contained in a single circular chromosome (recall that humans have twenty-three pairs of X-shaped chromosomes). However, bacteria can also have isolated genes, independent of the chromosome, which they frequently obtain through exchanges with other bacteria. These 'extra' genes are called *plasmids* and they are very important in infections. Plasmids allow bacteria to acquire new capabilities, for example resistance to an antibiotic, or generating a lethal toxin, as happens in the cases of diphtheria and cholera. Other diseases caused by bacteria are tuberculosis and plague.

Viruses: the smallest life form?

The first signs of the existence of microorganisms smaller than bacteria date back to the 1870s when some Dutch scientists realized that there were mysterious agents that could pass through the filters that held back bacteria and, having done so, cause infections. The first virus was described in 1898 and, since then, more than 5,000 different types have been identified. As with bacteria, it's believed that most of them haven't been discovered yet.

Viruses are the tiniest life forms in existence (between 100 and 500 times smaller than bacteria), although many people debate whether they are really alive or not, the reason being that they are not able to function alone because they must invade a cell in order to divide. In fact, viruses are nothing more than a group of genes surrounded by a more or less complex capsule that enables them to penetrate the cells of animals, plants or even bacteria themselves. Unlike the latter, they tend not to bring any benefit to the organisms they infect: they are more like parasites.

They are also the planet's most abundant organism and are found in all ecosystems. If we lined up all the viruses in the oceans, for example, they would extend 100 times further than the limits of our galaxy. Some are innocuous for humans and others can cause chronic (like hepatitis) or acute (like influenza or the common cold) diseases. Viral infections tend to be generalized and don't cause pain, unlike the bacterial kind, which are normally localized and cause inflammation or pain in the affected area.

However, viruses can be used to our advantage. They are essential, for instance, as tools in a great number of laboratory experiments. They enable us to introduce genes into cells, which can be useful not only in experiments but also for treatments like gene therapy. And, for quite some time now, viruses that attack bacteria (called *bacteriophages*) have been studied with a view to their use as an alternative to antibiotics.

Our current knowledge of genetics and molecular biology allows us to manipulate viruses in every conceivable way. In the opinion of the Galician virologist Luis Martínez-Sobrido, professor and head of a virology research group at the Texas Biomedical Research Institute in San Antonio (USA), 'there's no end to the possibilities'. He adds: 'In the last sixty years since Watson and Crick discovered the structure of DNA, more progress has been made in the study of living beings than in the entire history of humanity.'[1]

Certainly, for some years now we've been able to play with the genes contained in a virus, putting them in or removing them as we see fit, depending on whether the aim is to eliminate one of their functions or add a new one. One example is the use, in studies for the Ebola vaccine, of VSV, a virus that's inoffensive for humans, into which Ebola genes have been introduced in the hope that this will cause an immune response but without developing the disease. 'From the technical point of view, it's only a matter of time before we'll be able to do anything we want with viruses', says Dr Martínez-Sobrido. 'As they said in the film, *I Am Legend*, viruses are like cars. With a good driver at the wheel, a car will take us where we want to go, and we'll benefit from that. A bad driver, however, can cause death.'

But we also need to remember that studying viruses is complex and expensive, especially because of their size. In the words of Luis Martínez-Sobrido:

1   This and the following quotes are from an interview by the author with Luis Martínez-Sobrido [translation: JW].

We virologists are like astronomers. Both need big, expensive equipment to magnify very small and distant objects. Viruses are so tiny you can't see them with traditional microscopes. They require expensive, complex, electronic microscopes. Computer science is revolutionizing this field, but there's also a big economic cost. The same thing goes for the reagents that are necessary for cultivating and studying viruses. Nevertheless, the main limitation isn't economic resources but personnel. It seems that the adventurous, inquiring spirit has been disappearing lately, perhaps because our society values other qualities more than research or working to improve the quality of life. After all, the budget of a research laboratory is less than what many footballers are paid.

Viruses aren't only harmful because of the infectious diseases they cause. It's also been found that they play an important role in cancer. Some experts say that up to 20 per cent of cancers could have a viral cause, although at the moment only a few are known and the figure could be much higher in reality. For example, there's a relationship between certain kinds of hepatitis and liver cancer, between the retroviral infection HTLV-1 and leukaemia, and between the human papillomavirus and cancers of the uterus (which is why a vaccine was produced to protect women against the virus and, hence, cancer). It's also believed, as some studies suggest, that the onset of diabetes might be in some way related to previous viral infections. One theory ventures that certain viruses might force our defence systems to attack our own tissues, which would eventually destroy the pancreas cells that produce insulin.

Fungi: microscopic mushrooms

The third large group of microorganisms that cause major health problems are fungi. There are about 1.5 million different species, of which, once again, only a small part – 5 per cent – is known. Some 300 that are toxic for humans have been identified. In general, they are bigger and more complex organisms than bacteria or viruses. Most of them consist of sets of cells, but there are also some with just one cell. Many species of fungi are microscopic, but some are easily identifiable to the naked eye, for example mushrooms or those responsible for mould on food. Fungi also participate in processes of decomposition and fermentation and have been very important in the discovery of antibiotics, as I will explain below.

The fungi that cause diseases in humans are, in particular, of the genera *Aspergillus*, *Candida* and *Cryptococcus*. Fungus infections are unusual and are especially seen in immuno-compromised people, for example those suffering from AIDS. In such cases, they can even cause death. *Candida* are the fourth most common cause of blood infections in hospitals, with a 40 per cent mortality rate. Infections spread by *Aspergillus*, which are less common, kill in 80 per cent of cases. *Cryptococcus neoformans*, which left untreated can cause death, accounts for about a million fatalities worldwide every year, some 60 per cent in sub-Saharan Africa. It usually enters through the lungs and spreads rapidly around the whole body.

Fungi are especially resistant to treatment. There are only a few kinds of effective drugs (called *antifungals*) and some fungi have already developed resistance to them. A further problem when treating fungal infections is that it usually takes too long to diagnose them. It is necessary to wait until the fungi extracted from a patient grow in a special medium before they can be identified, a process that can take up to forty-eight hours, during which time the infection can worsen. New techniques are presently being studied with the aim of reducing this waiting time to a few hours.

2

The Story of a Never-Ending Struggle

It took us many centuries to discover that we were being killed by living beings we couldn't even see. In fact, we've been at the mercy of microorganisms for most of our history because we didn't have a good strategy for dealing with them. This is a struggle we were spectacularly losing until very recently. At least in developed countries, science has provided us with tools – which I will describe in the next chapter – that can end up holding many kinds of microbes in check. Furthermore, we now know the cause of almost all infectious diseases and how they are transmitted, which allows us to look for effective means of curbing them with social, health, hygienic and even urban planning interventions. In some extraordinary cases, we've achieved the total elimination of a microbe from the planet and it's possible that we will soon be able to repeat this feat with others. Despite this situation, which invites some degree of optimism, we shouldn't forget that, on numerous occasions throughout history, microbes have influenced our destiny as a species.

The invisible hand behind things

The fact is that microorganisms have played an extremely important role at crucial moments in the history of humanity. And vice versa. The fact that we've been evolving and constructing complex social networks has enabled infections to spread much more efficiently to reach every continent, which they might never have achieved without us. This parallel progress of humans and microbes began when our ancestors left their nomadic life and started living in settlements where they set about cultivating the land. As towns and cities grew bigger, more people lived in close proximity, sanitary conditions worsened and diseases spread more easily. Outside organisms, the chances of survival of microbes causing tuberculosis or leprosy, for example, are very slight, and they could therefore only start spreading contagion in any significant way when human beings started to live crammed together. Prior to this, it was difficult for these microbes to jump between small groups of people who lived in isolation from each other, which is why they never caused epidemics.

When they made the transition from hunters to farmers, humans also came to share their living space with domesticated animals. It is believed that this made it easier for many microbes to jump from one species to another. For example, diseases as widespread as smallpox, mumps, diphtheria, measles and whooping cough are caused by microorganisms that, in all likelihood, originally came from animals. In the coming chapters, we will see that this is also true for the more recent pandemics.

We have no record of any epidemic until the classical Greco-Roman period when there were three known major plagues. The plague of Athens (of 430 BCE, the oldest epidemic on record) broke out after the inhabitants of nearby towns fled to the city to seek protection from the Spartan advance. The terrible conditions of hygiene in overcrowded Athens allowed the epidemic, perhaps smallpox, to spread unchecked. A quarter of the population died of the plague, eventually giving victory to Sparta in that war, which is why it's said that, in some sense, a microbe hastened the end of the golden age of Greek culture.

The second major epidemic of the period is that known as the Antonine plague, which hit the Roman Empire in 166 CE. It probably originated in Seleucia (about 30 kilometres southeast of modern Baghdad) and is also thought to have been smallpox. It marked the beginning of the decline of Rome, which was completed with the third great disaster, the Justinian plague, in Constantinople in 542 CE. Apparently caused by the bacterium *Yersinia pestis*, it lasted for a year, followed by two whole centuries of new outbreaks, and it is thought to have killed a total of 100 million people.

A few centuries later, during the Crusades, the Christian attacks often failed owing to epidemics of dysentery, typhoid fever or smallpox, diseases the crusaders brought back from foreign lands to their countries of origin in Europe. The opening up of trade routes between Asia and Europe, thanks to the efforts of Marco Polo in the thirteenth century, also made it easier than ever before for microbes to travel between continents. Indeed, most infectious diseases had spread everywhere by the Middle Ages.

It's all too well known that infections played a key role in the Europeans' victory over the indigenous peoples of the Americas in the fifteenth and sixteenth centuries. People in the New World had never suffered from many diseases like smallpox or measles which were common in Europe. It's believed that the reason why these infections didn't exist in the Americas is that, there, human beings had few domesticated animals, which, as I've said, were the origin of

Just one victim, tremendous consequences

History has also changed thanks to the premature disappearance of some important figures. For example, Ramses V died of smallpox in 1157 BCE just before his 30th birthday. The leader Pericles, who was eminent enough to have given his name to a whole century of Greek culture, died in the Athens epidemic of 430 BCE. The death of Alexander the Great from an unknown infection in 323 BCE at the age of 33 brought about the fall of his great empire. King Alfonso XI of Castile died in a Black Death epidemic when fighting against Arabs in Gibraltar. Smallpox, which largely wiped out the English Stuart dynasty, also claimed as victims other European monarchs, among them Louis I of Spain, Louis XV of France and Peter II, Tsar of Russia.

many of the European epidemics. In the Americas, people coexisted mainly with ducks, llamas and alpacas, which are not major microbe reservoirs. So, these indigenous peoples had no immunity whatsoever against any of the new pathogens brought in by the invaders, and they began to die in huge numbers as soon as contacts were made. However, the exchange wasn't wholly unidirectional. It's believed that the conquistadors took home to Europe other diseases like syphilis and typhus.

In the 120 years after Christopher Columbus arrived in the Americas, about 90 per cent of the indigenous populations died, more because of infection than war. For example, fifty years after Hernan Cortés landed in Mexico, the population had fallen from 30 million to 3 million. Cortés's victory in the siege of Tenochtitlan in 1521 was possible after only seventy-five days because a smallpox epidemic devastated the city. Apart from his superior arms, the victory of Francisco

Pizarro over the Inca empire in 1531 is also thought to have been due to smallpox. This is also why just over 160 men were able to defeat Atahualpa's army of more than 80,000 soldiers, much to the surprise of both sides.

This difference of immunity between Europe and America, not only defined the future of the continent but also led to the enslavement of whole peoples. The victorious Europeans soon realized that they didn't have a big enough workforce available, so they resorted to 'importing' slaves. Nearly 20 million people from West Africa were abducted and borne off to the New World. So, the whole history of black culture in the Americas began because of deadly epidemics set off by the European conquistadors. This traffic also meant that still other diseases like yellow fever were introduced into the Americas.

A bacterium to blame for a new religion

Some theories hold that an infection might have been the cause of the founding of the Anglican Church. Henry VIII was having problems fathering children with Catherine of Aragon, possibly because he'd had syphilis some years earlier. Since Catholic doctrine wouldn't permit his divorce, he decided to create a new church with its own rules, including one that said that marriage didn't have to be for life. So, a bacterium could have been responsible for the changes in sixteenth-century European morality which led to puritanism.

The French tried to construct a canal in Panama in 1880, but a yellow fever epidemic thwarted the project for almost twenty years. In the end, it was finally achieved by the United States in 1913 once the yellow fever was under control. The same disease had killed 10 per cent of the inhabitants of New

York at the beginning of the eighteenth century. In 1802, the French army in Haiti lost a good number of its men, including the general, to yellow fever, which made it easier for the slaves to win the island's independence.

Microbes have fortuitously played a part in many historic decisions. For example, the army of Charles VIII of France had to discontinue its occupation of Naples at the end of the fifteenth century because of a syphilis epidemic, which was more severe in those days than the form of the disease that has survived until the present day. Other diseases like typhus have determined the results of entire wars, for instance when the defeat of the French army prevented Napoleon from conquering the whole of Europe. In fact, it's believed that, in most wars until the middle of the twentieth century, more people died because of infections than as a direct result of combat.

Rats, fleas, and bacteria

On the list of history's worst epidemics, plague has a prominent place. It's caused by *Yersinia pestis*, a bacterium that lives in rats, which have fleas, and is transmitted to humans by flea bites. It can cause inflammation of lymphatic nodules, forming the typical tumours called *buboes* (hence the name bubonic plague). Another type can also bring on a general infection and kill in a few hours. A third kind mainly affects the lungs and, left untreated, causes death in 100 per cent of cases. Nowadays, it's not such a serious disease, as we have a vaccine and antibiotics that can eliminate the bacterium in most cases but, even so, we can't claim that it's been eradicated. At the beginning of this century, for example, more than 2,000 cases of plague were still being diagnosed worldwide, most of them in Africa.

Delayed benefits

In the seventeenth century, the small town of Eyam, in the heart of England, was devastated by the Black Death. It's believed that the disease came from London, in a flea-ridden bundle of cloth. When the townspeople realized what was happening, they closed themselves in their houses to avoid contagion, but it was too late. By the end of the epidemic, 259 of the town's 350 inhabitants had died.

A few centuries later, Eyam found a way to benefit from this dark episode in its history, by organizing tours of the town and describing all the grisly details of how the plague nearly wiped it off the map.

There have been three significant epidemics of plague: the Justinian plague, that of the Middle Ages, which I've already mentioned, and one that broke out in Asia in the nineteenth century and has lasted through to the present day. But plague has almost certainly been with us for millennia. We can find descriptions of what sounds like the bubonic plague in the Bible and, specifically, in the First Book of Samuel, which speaks of the sickness that afflicted the Philistines because they'd captured the Ark of the Covenant. But when the thieves, terrified by what they believed was divine wrath, returned the Ark to its rightful owners, the plague also spread among the Jews, which goes to show that bacteria don't understand religions.

The most serious plague epidemic was the one in the mid-fourteenth century that raged across all of Europe, Asia and North Africa. Known as the Black Death or the Pestilence, it killed 25 million people, or half the population of the affected continents. The epidemic began in Asia and spread throughout Europe in just three years. The practice of *quarantine* (isolating a person who's suspected of being infected) dates precisely from this period. There were several outbreaks of Black Death in Europe until it was seen for the last time in the seventeenth century in the north of the continent, and in the eighteenth century in the south.

The bacterium responsible for plague wasn't discovered until the nineteenth-century epidemic that hit China. In 1894, Alexandre Yersin and Shibasaburo Kitasato independently identified it in Hong Kong. The Swiss Yersin was having problems in studying the disease as he wasn't permitted to examine the bodies of the victims, which were all being sent to Kitasato's laboratory. At the time, the latter, an eminent microbiologist, especially well known for his work with Robert Koch on tuberculosis and tetanus, was the clear preference of the authorities. By contrast, Yersin received no support, but he wasn't discouraged by that. He built a thatched hut, which became his laboratory, and started bribing morgue workers to give him access to the victims. Despite all the difficulties, Yersin ended up with the fame, partly because of errors in Kitasato's work. Yersin decided to name the new microbe *Pasteurella pestis* in honour of Pasteur but, years after his death, the name was changed to *Yersinia* in recognition of his contribution.

As I've said, plague is far from being a thing of the past. For example, there was an outbreak in China in early August 2009. It was a pneumonic plague and, by the time it was made public, ten people were infected and two had died. The authorities immediately quarantined 10,000 people to stop the contagion from spreading.

The 'Spanish' flu

The first known influenza pandemic is that of 1580 and, since then, there have been about thirty major outbreaks. In the twentieth century, for example, there were four: in 1900, 1918, 1957 and 1968. The pandemic of 1918 deserves special mention, as the last major health catastrophe of the twentieth century to affect the whole world – at least until the onset of AIDS. In terms of the number of victims, it's considered to rank third among the pandemics (after the Black Death of the Middle Ages and the smallpox that exterminated most of America's indigenous peoples).

Although the 1918 pandemic is traditionally called 'Spanish flu', the part of the globe where it began isn't known for sure. Spain was the first country to report cases – hence the name. In the debate about its origins, the main suspects are France, the United States, Spain itself and some countries of Asia. The final death toll isn't clear either. The figures range from 20 to 100 million people, according to different studies or, in other words, up to ten times more than the number of people who died in the First World War. This could signify between 2 per cent and 5 per cent of the total population of the planet (of which possibly 50 per cent was infected), with particularly high rates among people aged between 25 and 45.

Oddly enough, rather than being directly caused by the influenza virus itself, most deaths were the result of pneumonia brought on by bacteria. The virus would have broken through the physical barriers protecting the airways, thereby allowing the bacteria, which are normally on the surface and don't cause problems, to get inside tissues and end up causing deadly infections. It's thought that this is partly why the death tolls of the 1957 and 1968 pandemics were much lower (100,000 and 700,000 respectively), because antibiotics to fight secondary bacterial infections were then available to everyone, while they didn't exist in 1918. The treatments recommended then didn't go beyond leeches (to suck blood, which was thought to balance the body 'humours') or rubbing with menthol, both of which were clearly useless.

Sometimes pandemics have sneaky beginnings. In this case, for example, the first flu outbreak in January 1918 was mild and nobody regarded it as being more serious than a normal flu. By spring that year, it was already crossing the United States, but still no one paid much attention. Meanwhile, in Europe, fully embroiled in the First World War, it was starting to be a more serious problem. That summer, a second outbreak, more serious than the first one, began in Switzerland and reached American shores in September that year. Most cases were clustered in October and November, but a third wave was to appear early in 1919, followed by a fourth and final minor one in the spring of 1920.

The pandemic worsened because of mismanagement by the authorities, a state of affairs that has kept recurring throughout history, to this very day. For example, the US government's tactic was to downplay it. President Woodrow Wilson didn't make a single declaration about the situation. The authorities asserted that there was no reason to be alarmed if proper precautions were taken. The government said it didn't want the population to feel demoralized because 'fear kills more people than the disease', as a public health commissioner in Chicago put it. The aim was to make Americans believe that the pandemic was nothing worse than seasonal flu. Yet the symptoms were very different. Some infected people died within twenty-four hours, bleeding from their eyes and ears. The number of victims was rising by the day, but the authorities kept insisting that the outbreak was ending. The effect was exactly the opposite of what they hoped for: people in the United States lived in a state of fear, unable to trust the media and attentive only to rumours. They stopped going to work, shops closed, and the transport, food distribution, shops, medical treatment and communication systems all broke down. Only a few cities, San Francisco among them, decided to break the code of silence and alert the population in order to avoid total collapse.

We don't learn from our errors

The organizational problems that aggravate the effects of a pandemic today are less common, but they still exist. The dithering of many leaders in 2020 when faced with the beginnings of the COVID-19 pandemic would be an example of this. Nevertheless, it's been worse on other occasions. With the onset of the 2003 SARS epidemic, the Chinese government concealed the outbreak, thus causing panic in the cities because of lack of information and feelings of mistrust. The same thing happened in the early days of the bird flu outbreak when the governments of Thailand and Indonesia concealed information. And during the 2009 swine flu outbreak, even though the data flowed fast and clearly in most parts of the world, in countries like Argentina, the attempts of politicians to cover up the gravity of the situation contributed towards increased levels of contagion.

The response in Spain was not unlike that in the United States. Although it was the first country to recognize publicly that it had been hit by an epidemic, this didn't happen until five months after its onset. By then it was too late to stop it. The only solution was to hide. People protected themselves by covering their faces with handkerchiefs and locking themselves away in their houses. The dead were unceremoniously buried in mass graves for fear of contagion, a task the army frequently had to deal with as the citizens were unwilling to do it. In the villages, churches were forbidden to toll the death knell in order not to further demoralize the population, and life was all but paralysed for several months. The government had little idea of what measures to take, as was demonstrated by the fact that the beginning of the school year was delayed in order to prevent gatherings in classrooms, but crowd-pulling shows weren't banned. In Barcelona, even when the governor finally decided to cancel the main public events scheduled for that autumn, the Swiss founder of Barça, Joan Gamper, demonstrating that the threat wasn't taken seriously enough, decided to ignore this precautionary measure and to go ahead with the first match of the Catalonia championship, with the excuse that it would be in the open air with minimal risk of contagion.

The resuscitated virus

In 2005, a group of scientists, including Adolfo García-Sastre, a Spanish virologist working at the Mount Sinai Hospital, New York, managed to read the genome sequence of the virus that caused the 1918 flu pandemic. The biological material was taken from a well-conserved frozen corpse found in the glaciers of Alaska. The genetic information they obtained allowed them to re-create the virus in the laboratory and, with this synthetic virus, to reproduce the lethal effects of the infection in mice. The aim was to understand how the 1918 virus functioned and why it had been so deadly, in the hope of being able to design better drugs and vaccines against future pandemics.

With these experiments, for example, it was possible to confirm that this virus multiplied 40,000 times faster under laboratory conditions than the ones we see today. Prior to this, there were two nonexclusive theories to explain why the pandemic had been so devastating. One was that the virus had been more aggressive than other strains, and the new results demonstrated that this was so. The second was that there was a special predisposition in the population – and not only due to problems deriving from the war – which included malnutrition and poor public health facilities. But this possible susceptibility is hard to demonstrate, as there isn't enough material conserved for carrying out studies.

The work of Dr García-Sastre and his colleagues aroused the fears of both citizens and other scientists who believed that it would be dangerous to 'resuscitate' such a terrible virus. Others believed that the chances of the new virus escaping weren't very high, while the authors of the study argued that the benefits greatly outweighed the possible risks. Naturally, the safety measures around people handling these kinds of microbes are exhaustive, and accidents are therefore unlikely. Moreover, it's believed that today's population has more immunity to the virus than people did in 1918 because, since then, the circulation of variants similar enough to the original one might have generated a certain response that could protect us. The virus has been studied ever since that time without any notable incident.

Smallpox, a disease of the past

There is only one microbe causing diseases in humans that we have managed to eradicate from the planet. This sole example, so far, is the virus responsible for smallpox, a disease characterized by a generalized rash with fever and which, in serious cases, can have a mortality rate of between 20 and 60 per cent. It also has numerous sequelae, including blindness.

It is believed that, throughout history, the smallpox virus has killed more humans than any other, and not only in ancient times. In the eighteenth century, 400,000 Europeans died of smallpox every year and, in the twentieth century, it killed between 300 and 500 million people worldwide. In 1967 alone, it infected up to 15 million people, according to a World Health Organization (WHO) report.

The success in terms of healthcare has been due to vaccination campaigns which, as I will explain below, began in the nineteenth century. The last smallpox patient was registered in the United States in 1949, while the world's last natural infection was seen in Somalia, in 1977. Vaccinations which, in themselves, could give rise to small outbreaks of smallpox, ceased to be given not long afterwards. In May 1980, the 33rd World Health Assembly officially declared the world free of smallpox.

Poliomyelitis: next on the list?

Poliomyelitis, more simply known as polio, is a disease that causes paralysis in 1 per cent of those afflicted by it because the virus responsible destroys nerves. The most frequent kind is paralysis of the legs, but if the nerves controlling the muscles related with breathing are affected, it can be fatal. Some kinds of paralysis reverse in the first year but, after that time, few improve. It's calculated that, at the beginning of the twenty-first century, between 10 and 20 million people had survived polio, with varying degrees of sequelae. In 90 per cent of cases there are no symptoms.

The disease was discovered in 1840 and the virus that causes it, the poliovirus, in 1908. It's mainly contracted through water contaminated with faeces of infected people (where the virus can live for weeks), although saliva can also be a source of transmission. The number of cases of polio increased spectacularly at the beginning of the twentieth century, which spurred on the quest to find a vaccine. Jonas Salk achieved the first (1952) and Albert Sabin the second (1962). In 1988, there were 350,000 cases of polio in the world. It was initially expected that the disease would be eradicated by 2000, but that didn't happen. In 2007, there were 1,315 cases recorded and, in 2008, another 1,643; despite everything, this was a remarkable decline in just twenty years. The year with the fewest cases was 2001: just 483 were recorded. Progress seems to have stalled a little since then.

Since the turn of the century, $6,000 million have been spent on preventing and controlling polio. In early 2009, a new initiative was announced to eliminate it from the few places where it still exists (especially Nigeria, India, Afghanistan and Pakistan) and thereby to make it history's second eradicated disease. An investment of $630 million was made, donated by the Bill & Melinda Gates Foundation, Rotary International groups and the governments of Germany and the United Kingdom, which was distributed by the Global Polio Eradication Initiative (GPEI), part of the WHO. The strategy was mainly to increase vaccination of small children, as this is the most effective preventative. Although the hoped-for results haven't yet been completely achieved, the experts are optimistic and believe that there is every chance that polio will end up disappearing altogether.

Of the three existing variants of poliovirus, type 1 is the most aggressive. In 1999, type 2 was eradicated. Only a few samples were kept for study or continued production of vaccines. This might have been recorded as the second microorganism to be eliminated from the planet if it weren't for the fact that, in 2005, it made a surprise reappearance in the middle of Africa. By 2008, it had resulted in thirty cases of paralysis and, by the middle of 2009, a further hundred,

Titbits: famous people with polio

Here are some of the famous people who suffered from poliomyelitis. Many of them survived without visible sequelae:

Alan Alda	Arthur C. Clarke
Francis Ford Coppola	Joe Dante
Donovan	Ian Dury
Mia Farrow	Mel Ferrer
Frida Kahlo	Jack Niklaus
Joni Mitchell	Itzhak Perlman
Doc Pomus	Walter Scott
Donald Sutherland	Neil Young

The most famous polio patient in history, the president of the United States, Franklin D. Roosevelt, was most probably confined to a wheelchair because of another disorder, the Guillain-Barré Syndrome.

together with the possibility that it would start spreading to other areas. The origin of these new outbreaks was the vaccine that was supposed to eliminate it.

This happens because the vaccine that is presently being used is the so-called OPV (oral polio vaccine), the one discovered by Sabin. It is very effective. The problem is that it's made from attenuated viruses and it's known that, in some cases, they revert to their active form, recover their aggressiveness and cause spontaneous outbreaks. Although it is relatively rare (seen in just one case among almost 8 million vaccinated people), this is precisely what occurred in 2005 with the vaccine against the type 2 virus. In 2009, there were 124 cases of paralysis in Nigeria caused by this vaccine.

Some critics believe that, because of this potential danger, polio will never be wholly eradicated as long as the OPV vaccine is being administered. Hence, in developed countries, another vaccine is used, namely the IPV vaccine discovered by Salk, which is made from a form of the virus that is unable to reactivate. IPV is more expensive and dangerous to produce (and made only in places where security measures are of a high standard) and, moreover, it must be injected, which means it's less appropriate in poor countries. Scientists are still looking for an improved vaccine that would combine the best features of both OPV and IPV.

The main reason that polio is still around is the difficulty of vaccinating the entire population. In Nigeria, for example, the vaccination of children in the Islamic states of the north was halted for a while because of a rumour that the vaccine caused both infertility in women and AIDS. The most conservative religious leaders recommended that the population should not be vaccinated, and the upshot was that there were major outbreaks of polio in the country, after which the virus spread, first to neighbouring states, and then to twenty other countries that had already eliminated the disease, some of them as far away as Indonesia. Nigeria itself accounted for more than half the world's new cases of poliomyelitis.

However, in September 2020 it was announced that Africa was finally free of the polio virus (the wild version: there are still vaccine-derived cases, as described above). The last case of the disease on the continent was recorded in Nigeria in 2016. While science provided an effective vaccine that eliminated polio in most countries, clearing the African continent of the virus is actually a triumph of thousands of health and social workers and campaigners who have fought tirelessly over the years to ensure that the vaccination programmes worked, despite all the obstacles. Without their commitment, this would have never been possible.

But polio still exists in the world. It remains in Afghanistan and Pakistan, where the vaccines didn't reach war-torn zones to which neither the UN nor the WHO had access. In Pakistan, extremist leaders have proclaimed fatwas against vaccinators, claiming that the vaccine isn't safe. In India, the problems are mainly overcrowding and poor hygiene, which facilitates transmission of the virus. Until these obstacles are overcome, total eradication of polio won't be feasible.

Cost in lives, cost in money

It is calculated that infections have a very high economic cost owing to the consequences both of their mortality and the temporary or permanent disability they cause. This is easier to see in certain epidemics or pandemics. For example, the 1994 outbreak of plague in India caused a massive exodus of 0.5 million people, together with the closing of factories and, logically, a reduction of tourism in the country. It's estimated that the cost of this was $2,000 million. The 1991 cholera epidemic in Peru paralysed not only tourism but also the fishing industry, as all fish exports were stopped. The losses amounted to some $775 million. The 2003 SARS epidemic cost Asia $140,000 million, mainly due to the decline in tourism. We don't yet know what the cost will be of having paralysed the world economy for some months because of COVID-19, but it too is expected to be thousands of millions of dollars.

But epidemics don't have to affect humans in order to have a major social and economic impact. Recall that the United Kingdom lost about $6,000 million as a result of the bovine spongiform encephalopathy (BSE) outbreak in the 1980s and 1990s (aka mad cow disease), which put an end to meat exports for several years.

In cases of endemic diseases, the calculations become

complicated. For example, it's believed that the economic losses because of AIDS in some African countries could amount to as much as a third of their gross domestic product. Tuberculosis causes annual losses of around $12,000 million. A 1995 study showed that countries where malaria is endemic have incomes that are 33 per cent lower than those of countries where the disease is absent, with a GDP loss of 15 per cent.

All of this demonstrates that infectious diseases have a major impact on diminishing a country's wealth, so finding a way to eliminate them is an important strategy, not only for saving lives but also for reducing poverty and assisting developing countries.

3

Our Arsenal

For thousands of years, the only defence we've had against infections has been our own immune system, a complex, highly effective mechanism that has enabled us to survive continuous invasions since the day of our birth. Unfortunately, there are limits to our immunity and, accordingly, microbes have been the leading cause of mortality in the human species for a long time.

It should be recalled that the average life expectancy of the first humans was about 25–30 years, with a very high infant mortality rate of 150–250 for every 1,000 births (the present figure is between three and ten per 1,000 in developed countries). Much of the blame lay with microorganisms because, without proper hygiene measures, antibiotics or vaccines, catching certain kinds of infection was a death sentence. In those days, growing old was very unusual. Instead of improving with progress, as might be expected, the figures kept getting worse, at least until the Middle Ages when life expectancy hit all-time lows. As I said above, this can be explained

by the fact that people were living in ever-larger cities without proper sanitation management, which fast-tracked the
spread of all infectious diseases.

It wasn't very long ago that all this changed radically.
Indeed, we can't claim to have found a way of dealing with
microbes until well into the twentieth century. In the United
States, for example, life expectancy was 47 years in 1900,
rising to 71 by 1970. In 1900, of every 100,000 people who
contracted an infectious disease, 797 of them died; in 1980,
the figure was only 36. Life expectancy not only doubled in
the twentieth century, but, as a consequence, the world's
population increased fourfold.

How were we able to overcome this very low 'expiry date'
that humans seemed to have by default? The most spectacu-
lar improvement is the result of having identified the causes
of infectious diseases. From the moment that we realized
that we were highly susceptible to invisible organisms, we
started looking for the means to bring them under control.
In this regard, introducing minimal hygiene measures such
as a good system for keeping sewage and drinking water
well separated was one of the essential steps, and it had a
more immediate impact. Another was slowly constructing
an arsenal to thwart the microbes by attacking them from
several angles. Over the past 100 years, we have learned to
produce vaccines, antibiotics and antivirals that have given us
a definitive advantage over microorganisms. In this chapter,
I will give an account of some of these weapons that are so
important for our survival.

Simple but vital

As I said, the advance that has had the greatest impact on
human health is quite simple and hasn't required exhaustive

scientific research: an improvement in hygienic conditions, which includes making water potable, and establishing effective systems of waste disposal and good management of hygiene in hospitals. These are simple measures that seem obvious to us today, but they enabled our first victory over infections. They still need to be applied in many developing countries where, owing to their absence, life expectancy continues to be more like that of our ancestors. Currently, in the Central African Republic, it's 53.7 years, in Lesotho it's also 53.7, and in Chad, it's 54, to cite the three countries with the lowest figures. By comparison, the highest in the planet is in Japan: 84.5 years.

Recommendations for preventing epidemics begin with simple measures like careful handwashing, especially if food is being handled and, even more so, if there's been any contact with faeces. With this straightforward precaution, it is possible to reduce the presence of microorganisms on our hands by 50 per cent. It's necessary to remember to clean all surfaces with soap and disinfectant, especially in kitchens and toilets as these are the zones where most microorganisms can accumulate. As for food, we can also avoid many problems if it's properly conserved, because decomposition favours the growth of all kinds of microbes. Similarly, in principle, it is recommended not to eat raw eggs or to leave leftover food outside the refrigerator for more than two hours.

Measures at the level of urban planning started to be taken seriously in the second half of the nineteenth century, at a time when a cholera pandemic had spread around the globe. It was in London where, in 1854, the disease had been related with drinking water for the first time, when Dr John Snow deduced that the infectious agent was transmitted by water and not by air, as most people had believed. By means of scientific deduction, Dr Snow mapped the cholera cases and realized that they were grouped around a pump in

Broad Street, which was the only source of drinking water in that part of the Soho neighbourhood. He then discovered that the well had been dug near a cesspit that had contaminated the water. Snow managed to get the pump disabled, although the authorities were never willing to recognize that he was right. This is one of the early examples of how basic public health measures can save thousands of lives.

Around the same time, the Hungarian doctor Ignaz Semmelweis defined the basic principles of antiseptic measures that are now applied in all hospitals. Dr Semmelweis worked in the Vienna General Hospital and noticed that, in one of the maternity wards, there was a suspiciously high percentage of puerperal fever, a disease that affects women after childbirth. Also applying the scientific method, he deduced that the culprits were medical students who went straight to the maternity wing without washing their hands after they had been handling cadavers and carrying out autopsies. Once the necessary hygienic measures were introduced, the cases of fever dropped dramatically, thus demonstrating that the students had unwittingly been contaminating the birthing mothers with microbes from the corpses.

When Semmelweis published his observations in 1847, they were ignored and ridiculed by his colleagues, who couldn't admit that a simple measure like handwashing could have such a major impact on health. Decades went by before it was recognized that he was right, after which his suggestions were applied in all hospitals. Unfortunately, Semmelweis died in a mental hospital, where he had been admitted after confronting the whole medical establishment of the city. He didn't live to see how his discoveries saved thousands of lives.

Pioneers like Snow and Semmelweis were essential in making it possible to design the first strategies for avoiding outbreaks of disease and epidemics once transmission by microbes was better understood. The next step was to find a way of helping our defences to deal with them.

The immune system

All organisms need to protect themselves from the microbes trying to invade them. Even bacteria themselves produce toxic substances against viruses that attack them. Plants and animals have more sophisticated mechanisms making up what we call the *immune system*.

The strong sex

It's been known for some time that there are significant differences between genders with regard to immunity. In spring 2009, a study on mice was published, showing that females have a stronger immune system than males. This is because female hormones, the oestrogens, join the battle against bacterial infections.

There are many things we don't yet understand about our immune system. For example, some studies show that too little sleep makes us more susceptible to colds. It's believed that if we don't sleep a minimum of seven or eight hours, disturbances appear in the production of substances that are necessary for the proper functioning of our defences.

Human defences consist of a network made up of tissues, cells, proteins and other substances that work together in perfect coordination to block anything detected as alien. Their way of acting is highly complex and, in fact, there are still many aspects we don't fully understand. To sum up, there's a first line of defence, the so-called *innate immune system*, which attacks the invader in a nonspecific way. The second phase, now more focused on each specific microbe, is called the *adaptive immune system*. Also participating in these responses is a type of blood cell called *leucocytes*, or WBCs (white blood cells), and *antibodies*, which are proteins that recognize specific parts of the microorganisms (known as *antigens*) and activate the cells capable of destroying them. The combination of all these factors means that, in most cases, we can manage to deal with any unwelcome organism quite quickly.

After an infection, the adaptive system retains the 'memory' of the microorganism it has defeated. This is triggered the next time we are faced by a similar danger, in such a way that our immune system responds faster and more effectively to ward off the disease caused by the microbe. This is the principle on which vaccination is based.

The next step forward: vaccines

The first effective treatment for stopping infections was vaccines. The English scientist Edward Jenner is responsible for having popularized the idea of activating the immune system before people are exposed to a virus that's responsible for a disease. This was at the end of the eighteenth century when smallpox was causing many deaths and complications in the United Kingdom. Jenner observed that women farmers who milked cows tended not to get infected with smallpox. Instead, many of them had a much milder form of the disease because they'd contracted cowpox, which was eventually found to be caused by a virus from the same family. Jenner correctly deduced that the first infection was somehow a protection against the more serious form. Indeed, we owe the word 'vaccine' (from cows) to

Jenner, who coined it from the Latin word *vaccinus*, which is derived from *vacca* (cow).

In 1796, in order to test his theory, Jenner took pus from a woman farmer with cowpox and inoculated an 8-year-old boy. Six weeks later, he tried to infect the boy with the human smallpox virus but failed as the child was resistant to the disease. This process was called *immunization*. It was later discovered that it happens because vaccinated people develop antibodies against the infectious agent to which they are exposed. The specific cells that produce them remain in the blood 'watching out' in case there's another invasion. If this occurs, they can quickly eliminate the microbe before it causes serious symptoms.

The trick of the vaccine, then, is that it can stimulate our defences without needing to make us ill. Jenner achieved this by using a close, but weaker relative of the microbe he wanted to block. Over the years, we've been discovering alternative ways of achieving the same results (see box opposite). Nowadays, many vaccines are made with the same microorganism that causes the disease, but it's killed or inactivated beforehand.

It must be recognized that the concept of immunization long predates Jenner. In China and India, similar procedures were being used some centuries before his time. There are books of Chinese medicine dating from as early as 1500 that describe them. One example is the story of a nun who lived on top of a mountain and believed she was the incarnation of a goddess with the mission of saving children. Her technique was preparing powders made of dried smallpox scabs and using a tube to blow them into the nostrils of small children, who then suffered a mild form of the disease but were thereby immunized.

We currently have effective vaccines against dozens of diseases, but some major ones are still lacking, for example

---

Types of vaccine

Vaccines are classified according to the material that's used to stimulate the immune response in our organism. This can range from a whole microbe (but making sure that it can't infect us) to only specific parts.

- With dead microbes: the microbe is killed and the whole 'corpse' is injected (as in flu, cholera and poliomyelitis vaccines).
- With 'attenuated' microbes: the microbes are made inactive before being injected, or less aggressive microbes from the same family are used (measles, mumps, rubella). This is the most common method.
- With proteins from the microbe: parts of the microbe able to induce an immune reaction but not the disease itself (hepatitis B, papilloma) are used.
- With 'toxoids': a toxin from a bacterium (the toxic substance that some of them secrete), which is attenuated by means of chemical or physical methods (tetanus, diphtheria).
- With 'conjugates': capsules that have some modified bacteria are used (*Haemophilus* influenza).
- Others: vaccines that use new technologies and that are not yet massively applied, so it isn't known how useful they will be. They can be synthetic, from DNA, using other viruses to introduce part of the microbe, etc. Many of the COVID-19 vaccines were based on these techniques.

---

for AIDS and malaria. The fact that childhood vaccination is mandatory in developed countries has enabled us to control many infections that once had terrible consequences, among them rubella, measles, mumps and poliomyelitis. The present vaccination schedule includes compulsory immunization (with some variations among countries) against diphtheria, tetanus and whooping cough (all three in a single vaccine called Tdap), measles, mumps (or parotitis) and rubella (the so-called triple viral vaccine, MMR), hepatitis A and B, *Haemophilus influenza*, flu, poliomyelitis, pneumococcus, rotavirus, chickenpox and meningococcus. The WHO has calculated that vaccines save between 2 and 3 million lives every year, especially among children who are particularly vulnerable to infections, since their immune system isn't fully developed.

There are also a few clever ways of heightening the effectiveness of vaccines, for example by including with them chemical substances called *adjuvants* that boost the vaccines for reasons that aren't always known. One of the most commonly used is alum, a compound substance based on potassium sulphate. And research is being carried out into alternative, more effective ways of administering vaccines – for example, using tattoo needles to inject them under the skin, or microneedle patches for transdermal delivery of protein crystals in order to avoid having to conserve the vaccine in the refrigerator, which is one of the main obstacles in attempts to get vaccines into remote areas or those with poor communications.

Being able to vaccinate the greater part of the population is essential for ensuring that there will be no transmission of infections, and thus no epidemics. This is why it is so important that everyone, without exception, should abide by the vaccination rules laid down by the experts. This leads to so-called *herd immunity*, which occurs when a high enough percentage of the population (at least 50 per cent but, better, 90–95 per cent) is immune to a disease. In these circumstances, it's impossible for a microbe to cause more than a localized outbreak simply because the people who can't get infected and, therefore, can't infect others, act as a barrier. Achieving herd immunity is what ensures that infectious diseases don't keep causing pandemics, and the most effective way of doing this is with vaccines.

Cancer vaccines

For some decades now, vaccines have been tested against other diseases, most notably cancer. Up to 20 per cent of cancers could be caused by microorganisms, especially viruses, although the exact figure isn't known. Many viruses integrate their DNA into the cells they invade, and this can activate oncogenes, the particular genes that cause cancer when they start functioning in an unregulated manner. Moreover, as they've evolved, viruses have developed proteins that deactivate the internal defence mechanisms of cells, many of which belong to the family of tumour suppressors that, apart from destroying an infected cell, also prevent it from turning cancerous. The classic example of this is the protein known as p53, which is a frequent target of viral proteins. Viruses then inadvertently disconnect the necessary protections that prevent cells from becoming malignant, thus increasing the risk of a tumour developing. Chronic infections like hepatitis can also create an environment conducive to cancer cells because the affected tissues produce substances that stimulate their growth, even though the initial attempt is to fix the lesion.

In most cancers, the possible carcinogenic microbes that cause them haven't yet been identified, but a few examples of their being discovered do exist. The best known of these is the human papillomavirus (HPV), which causes most cancers of the cervix and anus, as well as others of the vagina, mouth and penis, of which I will speak more in the next section. Moreover, it's suspected that HPV might also be related to lung cancers, while a virus called XMRV could cause some prostate cancers. The viruses causing hepatitis B and C and the bacterium *Helicobacter pylori* may, respectively, cause cancers of the liver and stomach. All of these diseases could some day, in principle, be prevented with vaccines.

The ability of vaccines to stimulate the production of antibodies has been harnessed to prevent diseases, but, in some cases, it can also be used to treat them. These are the so-called *therapeutic vaccines*. The type that is in the most advanced phase is also the one for cancer. The reason for this is that, for some time now, it's been known that immune system cells do much more than control infections. Another of their main functions is to get rid of cells in the organism that are starting to act dangerously. Hence, cells that could become cancerous are regularly eliminated, thus preventing the appearance of tumours. With age, this pro-tective mechanism seems to weaken for reasons that aren't yet clear, and the 'bad' cells end up finding ways to get around it. If it was possible to reactivate defences against cancer, not only would we be prolonging this protection, but we might also even be able to destroy cancers that have already formed.

Therapeutic vaccines work like those used against infec-tions. They provide the tools that the white blood cells need to identify the cells that must be eliminated. The main differ-ence is that, this time, the cells are from the body itself and not invading microbes. If it is to achieve this, the immune system must be educated to recognize some of the proteins on the surface of cancerous cells and to mobilize an effec-tive response against them. The key to success is being able to select the most suitable protein. Since all kinds of cancer present a particular profile of proteins on the surface of their cells, it is highly likely that a specific vaccine will need to be designed for every one of them. The most important thing in these cases is to prevent cross-reactivity affecting healthy cells. Known as an autoimmune response, this can end up being fatal. After all, although the cancerous cell is abnormal, it's part of the organism and most of the proteins it presents on its surface are the same as those on healthy cells.

In keeping with this principle, proteins that appear in excess in certain cancers have been isolated, and it's been possible to produce antibodies that recognize them and activate cells of the immune system that can eliminate malignant cells. A first vaccine of this type, which has had some success in treating prostate cancer, is already on the market, though it isn't effective enough to cure the disease. Others are still in the study phase and genetic techniques are even being used to obtain personalized vaccines for each patient.

The papilloma vaccine, a controversial solution

As we've just seen, it's been known for some time now that the human papillomavirus is responsible for a good number of cases of cervical cancer. It is sexually transmitted, and very easily so, especially because, at first, it presents no symptoms at all. Between 80 and 90 per cent of all sexually active women are infected by this virus at some or other point in their lives, but only a very small percentage will suffer serious consequences. HPV invades the cells that line the uterus, which, with time, keep transforming and acquiring irregular characteristics. Cytologies (known also as Pap smears, in honour of their inventor, the Greek doctor Georgios Papanicolaou) are a good way of detecting these changes, which is why they are regularly carried out in gynaecological check-ups. It's therefore been possible to achieve a major reduction in the incidence of this cancer. In fact, 80 per cent of uterine cancers in developed countries are discovered in women who haven't had a Pap test in more than ten years. Elsewhere in the world, where having regular check-ups is an almost non-existent concept, this cancer is still a serious problem.

In 2006, a vaccine against the most aggressive forms of HPV, produced by the company Merck, was marketed for the first time. Some countries, like Spain or the United States, and up to eighty more, quickly incorporated it into the vaccination schedule, for use before women become sexually active. In 2007, GlaxoSmithKline (GSK) started marketing its version of the vaccine and, before the year ended, it was being used in Australia and Europe. The vaccines were hailed as a kind of revolution in the field of cervical cancer treatment, and the way of eliminating it for once and for all.

However, the HPV vaccine was controversial from the start. Certain religious groups opposed it because they believed it encouraged promiscuity among adolescents. Moreover, some scientists criticized the fact that it had been made mandatory in so many places, with the high economic and health costs the policy involved, when cervical cancer is a relatively infrequent disease in a lot of countries. They pointed out that regular gynaecological check-ups are proven to be sufficiently effective for preventing the appearance of tumours and that this practice should be promoted instead of using a vaccine. Some believe that the economic interests of the pharmaceutical companies could have played a major role in some political decisions, and have criticized the haste with which the vaccine has been imposed, as well as decrying the fact that the necessary experiments to demonstrate its safety haven't been carried out. Nevertheless, governments have argued that there are no problems with the vaccine, and that it has considerable potential for healthcare, which has been demonstrated with time.

A certain number of mostly slight secondary effects of this vaccine have been reported. In February 2009, cases of adverse reactions appeared in Valencia. Two girls, on two consecutive days, suffered seizures and loss of consciousness a few minutes after receiving a second dose of the vaccine. Vaccinations with the batch that was then being used were immediately stopped. These were among the first serious reactions to be seen in Europe, after more than a million doses had already been given in Spain. In the United States, the figures were higher: 24 million vaccinations and more than 13,000 reactions. But this is still a very small percentage and only 7 per cent of these reactions were considered to be serious.

It's important to note that it hasn't yet been possible to demonstrate a cause–effect relationship between the vaccine and any of the more severe reactions. It can only be said that the problems correlate with the period of vaccination, but this might not have been more than a coincidence. Since the results are positive and there are very few negative effects, mass vaccination programmes are continuing, and most doctors recommend following each country's vaccination plans. Although there's been some opposition, the introduction of the vaccine has occurred on a substantial scale with no major complications, and it's hoped that the number of cases of cervical cancer will fall dramatically around the world. For example, it's calculated that, at the present rate of vaccination, the disease could be completely eradicated in Australia in the next twenty years.

The danger of listening to the wrong people

Ever since the early days of vaccination, some people have been against it. The fact that complications appear (usually in a low percentage of cases) and that we are voluntarily being injected with microbes, however inoffensive we're told they are, gives rise to suspicions. Apart from possible

health reasons, some people also reject vaccines for religious or ethical motives, a stand that could even endanger
a whole country. I mentioned earlier the case of poliomyelitis in Nigeria; another example would be the campaign
in Stockholm in 1873 against smallpox vaccination. Some
people said it wasn't safe enough and wielded the argument
of individual freedom or the right to decide whether to have
it or not. The percentage of vaccinated individuals dropped
rapidly from 90 per cent to 40 per cent. Not long afterwards,
there was a terrible smallpox epidemic in the city, which put
an end to all doubts and led to the reestablishment of the
mandatory vaccination schedule.

Even today, there are voices speaking out against vaccines. In recent years, there has been a trend in favour of
suppressing certain mandatory vaccines for children, despite
the evident benefits they bring. This fad began with a single
scientific study that has been proven wrong, and amply so,
ever since it was first published. An unwonted media campaign in support of these anti-vaxxers, with the help of some
particularly fervent supporters, has done the rest.

The beginning of this trend can be traced back to Dr
Andrew Wakefield who, in 1998, presented results that, he
claimed, demonstrated that the triple viral vaccine (against
mumps, measles and rubella) was associated with autism.
He based his conclusions on a very small sample of twelve
patients, eight of whom seemed to have developed symptoms
related to autism shortly after being vaccinated. The article
appeared in *The Lancet*, one of the most prestigious medical
journals, and immediately raised a hue and cry in the media
around the world. It was logical: if a vaccine that was systematically given to all the children in the world could cause
autism, even if only in a very small percentage of cases, the
impact this might have was immense.

As always happens when someone presents a hypothesis,

More conspiracies

The case of Wakefield isn't the only one that has sparked controversy over a vaccine. In France, in the 1990s, multiple sclerosis was linked with the vaccine against hepatitis B.
In the United States, others have spoken about the harmful effects of thiomersal, which is used as a preservative in some vaccines. And, in the United Kingdom in the 1970s, a doctor claimed that the whooping cough vaccine caused neurological damage. In none of these cases has scientific evidence been produced to support such claims.

scientists around the world immediately set about testing whether or not it is true. Only a month after Wakefield's article was published, the first studies appeared stating that the data he had used were far from correct, and it soon became clear that there were fundamental errors in his study. Moreover, in the next ten years, no one managed to come to the same conclusions as Wakefield had.

The corroborated opinion of so many experts should have been enough to put an end to the matter. But this case was different. Wakefield's erroneous conclusions had taken on a life of their own. Parents of autistic children embraced his findings as the rational explanation of their children's problems and began intensive campaigns to stop vaccinations everywhere in the world. These initiatives were reported in the press as front-page news. Yet, when scientific articles rebutting Wakefield's conclusions began to appear, the self-same newspapers either paid little attention to them for years, or they relegated the story to some inconspicuous place. The scientific truth didn't reach the public as compellingly as it should have and, as a result, the misinformation kept snowballing.

The cause was constantly gaining followers, and had the support of personalities like Jennifer McCarthy, an American actor who has an autistic son. Every day, more ill-informed celebrities took up the cause and there were even television series telling stories about unscrupulous pharmaceutical companies that didn't care about children's health. Lack of confidence in the state and health services played its part in the fact that some parents ignored the experts and heeded the rumours. Eventually, many of them refused to allow their children to be vaccinated even though their doctors assured them there was no danger.

The real precedent

Part of the public's irrational fear of vaccines might come from a historical case of the vaccine against RSV (respiratory syncytial virus). This was given to a number of children in 1966, two of whom died, while the rest were not protected against the disease (in some cases, the injections actually made it even worse).

A study in 2008 blamed the failure of the vaccine on the fact that it was not given with adjuvants, substances that activate the immune system. Without them, the effect of the vaccine was the opposite of what was expected.

Adjuvants weren't known until 1966 and, so far, no effective vaccine against RSV has been found.

The consequences for public health were quick to appear. In 1998, there were only fifty-six cases of mumps in all the United Kingdom. In 2008, however, there were nearly 1,500 sick children, almost 300 times more in only a decade. In the United States, between 2007 and 2009, it was calculated that 47,500 children were infected, of whom 204 died, as a result of the decline in vaccinations. This trend has continued to the present with sporadic outbreaks that could easily have been prevented in some countries.

It should be recalled that although mumps, measles and rubella seem to be insignificant diseases, they are not exempt from serious consequences. Three out of every 1,000 children die from measles, a figure that's rising in developing countries because of a lack of quality healthcare. Complications, infrequent but terrible, include blindness and brain damage. Mumps can cause encephalitis and sterility. The WHO had calculated that measles would be eradicated by 2010 but, thanks to Wakefield, that hasn't been possible. And this is why Europe is one of the industrialized zones with the highest numbers of cases of measles and, for example, is well ahead of South America, where it's been found that recent cases of measles came precisely from the Old Continent.

In the United Kingdom, the vaccination figures have varied, with periods when they've reached only 78 per cent of children (and, surprisingly, the figure has dropped to just 50 per cent in the London area). This is a long way from the 90–95 per cent that's needed for herd immunity. Although this figure had almost been attained in the 1990s, the situation this century is a big step backwards that will take time to correct. For similar reasons, there was a major outbreak of measles in the United States when, in 2000, it was considered that the disease had been eradicated in the country. In Minnesota, some cases of meningitis caused by *Haemophilus influenza B* were declared in 2008, although a vaccine had been available for this infection since 1993, and one of the children of anti-vaxxer parents ended up dying. Similar examples keep recurring from time to time.

Eventually, the press started paying attention to the numerous data refuting Wakefield's findings. In 2004, an article was published in *The Sunday Times*, demonstrating that there were irregularities in the way Wakefield had chosen patients for his work. Channel 4 broadcast a report on the subject the same year. The BBC followed suit in 2005, taking as its source a much more accurate and exhaustive study than Wakefield's, in which it was clearly demonstrated that there was no relationship between the vaccine and autism. Moreover, it was discovered that Wakefield had received money from lawyers who were preparing a lawsuit against vaccine manufacturers, and that he himself was trying to take out a patent on an alternative vaccine. Finally, the editors of *The Lancet* issued a statement acknowledging that there were inexcusable errors in Wakefield's article and, if they had known in time, these flaws would have been sufficiently serious to prevent its publication. Not long afterwards, the coauthors of the original article distanced themselves from the results and declared that they no longer supported Wakefield's theses.

It wasn't until 2009, five years after the press had recognized that the article was officially judged to be erroneous, that it was discovered that Wakefield had directly falsified the patients' data. He'd described symptoms that the children didn't have and claimed that these had appeared just after the vaccine was given, even though the patients' records indicated that, in most cases, whatever symptoms they showed had appeared much later. As a result, Wakefield was accused of scientific fraud.

Although the evidence is abundant, clear and irrefutable, a false perception of the reality still persists among some members of the public. Some 25 per cent of Americans still believe that there's a relationship between the vaccine and autism. Wakefield's study has always had its fanatical followers. For example, in 2009 there was quite a hullabaloo in the United Kingdom because a radio announcer kept recommending that children shouldn't be vaccinated. Some scientists who tried to inform the public of the truth even

Dangerous decisions

In the summer of 2009, one of the board members of Autism Speaks (the private foundation that invests most money in autism research) resigned. He did so in order to report the fact that the foundation was funding new studies on the relationship between vaccines and autism. He was the second person to leave for this reason.

Autism Speaks was established in 2005 as an initiative of a former executive of the television channel NBC. It had an annual budget of $33 million allocated for research, 2 per cent of which was earmarked for studying vaccines. The dissidents said they'd been giving out an erroneous message to the population, and were thus supporting theories that were demonstrably false, while the directors claimed that the aim was precisely the opposite, and that it was necessary to continue with the research in order to convince people that the theories weren't correct.

received death threats. Online disinformation is partly to blame, as is the stubbornness of journalists who say they must present two sides of the story even when there's not a shadow of doubt that only one is true.

Experts agree that vaccines are among the best drugs we have, as they are highly effective and have few side effects, and it's important that everyone should know this. For example, the Spanish paediatrician Maria Arantxa Horga, a specialist in infectious diseases and head of clinical research in a pharmaceutical company in the United States, says that, 'none of these [anti-vaxxer] assertions has been proven to be true and there's no evidence to support them. Vaccines prevent more than 2 million deaths every year around the world, and the relationship between benefits and risks is clearly favourable.'[2] Cases like Wakefield's have at least meant that pharmaceutical companies are exerting tighter control over their products. Dr Horga also notes that 'more tests are being done to improve the quality of vaccines and to understand all the secondary effects involved'.

Future challenges

In January 2016, a group of experts published in *Science* magazine a list of ten vaccines that most urgently need to be developed. By order of gravity, the diseases that should be prevented are: Ebola, chikungunya, MERS, Lassa fever, Marburgvirus, paratyphoid fever, schistosomiasis, Rift Valley fever, SARS and ancylostomiasis, all of them caused by viruses except for paratyphoid fever and ancylostomiasis. There's no treatment for any of them and, in many cases, they are fatal. I will discuss some of them shortly. Viruses like Ebola and Marburg haemorrhagic fever, which have recently caused serious problems, are among the main objectives. At the end of 2016, it was found in clinical trials that the rVSV-EBOV vaccine gives protection from Ebola in more than 70 per cent of cases and, although its effectiveness must still be thoroughly tested, it's starting to be administered as an emergency measure to part of the at-risk population in Guinea and Congo, in order to curb the latest outbreaks, which were threatening to spread throughout Africa.

However, vaccines that are effective against some of the infectious diseases with the most serious impact today, like AIDS and malaria, haven't yet been found. Another challenge

2   This and the following quotes are from an interview by the author with Maria Arantxa Horga [translation: JW].

Four questions for Adolfo García-Sastre, director of the Global Health and Emerging Pathogens Institute at the Mount Sinai Hospital in New York

What infectious diseases are most likely to cause serious pandemics in future?
There can always be a virus that might surprise us. For example, nobody imagined that a virus like HIV would cause a pandemic, which is still happening. Yes, it's known that flu gives rise to regular pandemics every ten to fifty years, but it's impossible to anticipate the severity.

So, how can we prepare for the next flu pandemic?
It's very difficult because of its unforeseeable nature. In order to prevent a flu pandemic, it's necessary to have vaccines that protect against more strains, and ideally against any strain of the flu virus.

Will it be possible to produce this universal vaccine some day?
The anti-flu vaccines we presently have aren't optimal. They don't give protection in a significant number of vaccinated people, the protection isn't lasting and, when it works, it only protects against the strains that are present in the vaccine. Since the strains of the circulating viruses change from one year to the next, and there are years when the strains in the vaccines don't match those that are circulating, you don't get good protection in these cases. More effective vaccines, covering more strains of the virus have been tested with animals but, long-term, highly expensive clinical trials with humans are needed to show whether or not they work.

Can other infectious diseases be eradicated thanks to vaccines, as happened in their day with smallpox and rinderpest?
Measles and polio, for example, are diseases that could potentially be eradicated with a suitable vaccine. But, in order to achieve this, we would need to be able to vaccinate more people than we do at present.

that has faced scientists for years is the universal flu vaccine. As we will see in Part Two, at present it's necessary to design a new one each season because the dominant strain changes from one year to the next, and the proteins on its surface are always different. A universal vaccine would recognise all forms of the virus, so a protein or part of the virus that varies very little should be used as a target. Finding this won't be easy but some candidates are already being studied, for example the least variable part of HA and NA proteins, which are being used to produce today's vaccines.

Antibiotics: the offensive begins

Apart from vaccines, the other important weapons in the struggle against microbes are antibiotics. It's difficult to say exactly when they were discovered. Traditional Chinese, Egyptian, Greek and Arab healers were using plants and fungi to treat infections centuries ago. Without knowing the mechanisms involved, the early doctors had discovered that there are substances in nature that block microbes. This would be the definition of *antibiotic*, a term used for the first time in 1942: any compound that kills a bacterium or inhibits its growth. Those used to battle viruses are called antivirals, and I will describe them below.

As early as 1877, the scientists Louis Pasteur and Robert Koch detailed how certain bacteria could interfere with the reproduction of others, a phenomenon they initially called *antibiosis*. It was clear that they were producing some kind of substance that had toxic properties for certain microbes. The first synthetic antibiotic, called arsphenamine (or Salvarsan, which was especially useful against syphilis) was obtained by the German physician Paul Ehrlich, also at the end of the nineteenth century. But Salvarsan had too many side effects to be used routinely with humans. The first commercially available antibiotic was Prontosil, which was discovered in 1932 in the Bayer laboratories by Gerhard Domagk, who, as a result, received the Nobel Prize in Physiology or Medicine in 1939. But the real revolution was ushered in by penicillin.

Alexander Fleming discovered penicillin in 1928 (see box), but at the time no one thought it could be of any

A classical story

Many people have heard or read about the accidental discovery of penicillin. On the morning of Friday, 28 September 1928, the Scottish scientist Alexander Fleming went to his laboratory in the basement of St Mary's Hospital, London, and saw that fungus had grown on a culture of bacteria that had accidentally been left open. Fleming had the reputation of being intelligent but very disorganized, a typical absent-minded genius, and this was his good fortune. Instead of throwing away the contaminated culture, he looked at it carefully and realized that there were no bacteria around the fungus. He deduced that the fungus, which was of the *Penicillium* genus, was producing some substance that was killing or curbing them, and he called it penicillin. It was thought that it could be useful as a disinfectant but not stable enough to be used in humans.

To be fair, it should be said that there were a number of forerunners who made discoveries similar to Fleming's but without leading to many practical results. The first scientific observations of fungi inhibiting bacteria date from 1870; by 1871, there was already discussion about the ability of *Penicillium* to suppress infections in humans; and, in 1875, the antibacterial activity of *Penicillium* was formally described in an article.

medical use. Ten years had to go by before Ernst Chain and Howard Florey revived Fleming's work. They saw that penicillin killed a significant variety of bacteria, but with few side effects. This meant that it was much more powerful than other similar drugs that were then being prescribed. In 1940, Florey and Chain published their first studies and Fleming, surprised that someone should be interested in his old discovery, decided to visit the scientists at their Oxford laboratory. Then, the surprise was on them. They didn't know that Fleming was still alive. Although they had worked independently, Fleming, Chain and Florey shared the 1945 Nobel Prize in Physiology or Medicine for their discovery.

Nevertheless, there was a major impediment to be overcome if the full potential of penicillin was to be taken advantage of: until a way of producing it in large purified quantities was found, it couldn't be used on a regular basis. This didn't happen until the 1940s, thanks to scientists working for the pharmaceutical company Pfizer, among others, and also the work of Dorothy Hodgkin (the first Englishwoman to be awarded a scientific Nobel) who determined the structure of penicillin using X-ray crystallography. It's rumoured that the relationship between Fleming, Chain and Florey wasn't particularly good, especially as Florey was irritated because the press gave Fleming most of the credit for the discovery when he believed that he'd done much more to ensure that the treatment reached the sick.

Penicillin was, then, the first antibiotic of relevant clinical use and it initiated the modern era of infection control. At present, there are twenty different kinds of antibiotics, each one with a specific use against certain kinds of bacteria. Some have severe side effects and are only used in special cases, while others are well tolerated and effective against the more common bacterial infections. The essence of a good antibiotic is that it attacks the bacterium but without affecting human cells, although this isn't always easy because many toxins are toxic for both.

Powerful poisons or a sophisticated messaging system?

Starting with penicillin, most antibiotics come from the same microorganisms that are found in the environment and, specifically, bacteria that live in the ground are the chief manufacturers. It was initially believed that the function of these substances was to kill other microbes and thus eliminate competition so that the bacteria that produced them could occupy an ecosystem. But another idea now being floated is that antibiotics could have more 'peaceful' functions – like communication, for example. After all, the microbes that produce them live surrounded by other microbes with similar needs and it's logical that they would be better off cooperating than fighting.

How might we humans have managed to turn a regular tool of communication among microorganisms into a substance that kills them? What we've done is merely to produce these substances in much greater quantities than those found in nature. In these high concentrations, they become toxic. It's deduced from this that if we use as treatment an antibiotic at doses below those that are harmful, the effect might be exactly the opposite, namely helping the microbes that are infecting us to communicate and reproduce better. And this could also play a role in the appearance of resistances.

Miracles with an expiry date

The great problem with antibiotics is that bacteria learn to survive them. Fleming himself predicted this in 1945. It's what he called *resistance*: a bacterium stops being susceptible to the drug that's normally used to kill it or inhibit it, and it's then necessary to find a new one that does the same job. And the guilty party is the very process that has enabled us to evolve to become the rational beings we are: evolution.

Resistance is nothing more than an example of natural selection. We know that the genomes of microorganisms are constantly accumulating small, spontaneous variations. As a simple statistical matter, it's possible that one bacterium out of the many millions that are exposed to treatment might have acquired one of these random variations in its genes, which would fortuitously make it immune to the drug. Evidently, a single bacterium can't do much. But it's necessary to think beyond that. While its poisoned peers are dying, the bacterium with the new 'power' survives and reproduces. Now we have two resistant bacteria, because the genes of the first one will also be passed on to its descendants. These bacteria will keep multiplying without problems. Still worse, the competition, or the bacteria that were still sensitive, would have been eliminated by the treatment so that, over time, we will have selected a resistant population originating from a single lucky bacterium. This explains the appearance of strains against which the usual drugs have no effect. The same weapon that protects us against bacteria is also the one that favours the strongest ones and helps them to replace the less aggressive ones.

Is there anything to be done against this side effect of antibiotics? Not much. Natural selection can't be stopped. But, yes, we can be careful. For example, we should use antibiotics only when necessary, and only those most indicated to combat the microorganisms responsible for each infection. Giving antibiotics 'just in case' only increases the possibilities of the existence of bacteria that become resistant. In many countries, this is clearly understood, and antibiotics can only be obtained with a prescription, and a prescription that doctors think twice about before giving it. In other places, however, the regulations are laxer.

This is why experts have long called for strict controls on the use of newer antibiotics in order to avoid making the same errors that have disabled the first generations of these drugs. It's also deemed important to educate the general public on the dangers of improper use of antibiotics. Self-medication with pills left over from a previous treatment, for example, tends to be incomplete, and this helps the bacteria to survive and acquire resistance.

The other thing we need to do at the same time is to keep looking for new drugs. This is how we've managed, so far, to keep infections under control despite resistances: by finding antibiotics that act differently and against which bacteria still have no defences. Within the time it takes for resistance to an antibiotic to appear, we can normally make a new one available. But the declining investment in antibiotics research, largely because of lack of interest among the pharmaceutical companies in a product that doesn't bring in big profits, has led us to the critical situation of the early twenty-first century where there are increasingly resistant bacteria and fewer treatment alternatives.

The microbes of the future

In 2000, the WHO recognized that the appearance of resistances could be the 'health catastrophe of tomorrow'. Indeed, a new generation of bacteria, which are almost impossible

Doctors fight resistance

Doctors can play a very important role in preventing the appearance of resistant bacteria. The first thing they must do is to prescribe antibiotics with caution and, if possible, only when it's confirmed that the patient has a bacterial infection. However, in the USA it's believed that 55 per cent of antibiotics are prescribed in cases where they are unnecessary and, frequently, it's the patients themselves who pressure the doctors to give them a prescription.

The doctor tries to choose the appropriate antibiotic and not to use by default the most powerful one on the market, as that would only favour the rapid appearance of resistances against the best antibiotics we have. The problem is, this can only be done when we know which bacterium is responsible and, in order to find out, it has to be cultivated in the lab, which is a process that can take days. In many cases, it's not possible to wait that long before starting a treatment. One solution is to begin with strong antibiotics and change to more specific ones when the diagnosis is known.

Finally, there are studies trying to ascertain if the number of days of treatment can be reduced. At present, treatment is continuous until several days after the symptoms disappear. Some experts believe that antibiotics only help the immune system to overcome the infection itself and, therefore, there's no need to prescribe them beyond the initial phases. According to these early studies, between one and three days would be sufficient for most of the usual infections.

to kill with any known drug, has recently started to appear. Will these bacteria begin to spread and replace their weaker relatives? Will we find the antibiotics capable of defeating them in time?

The real extent of cases of resistant bacteria around the world is still unknown. When the press speaks of outbreaks of 'killer bacteria' in a hospital, it's usually referring to these resistant bacteria. The most common among these is the methicillin-resistant *Staphylococcus aureus* (MRSA) which, impervious to most known antibiotics, first made its appearance at the end of the 1990s. In the United States, MRSA causes 100,000 infections every year, about 19,000 of which are fatal. This death toll is higher than that for AIDS. It has also been confirmed that up to 25 per cent of elderly people living in residences are infected by MRSA.

S. aureus is a bacterium with an impressive history of resistance. Only few years after penicillin was introduced in the 1940s, *S. aureus* bacteria were found that didn't respond. Their resistance was due to their ability to produce a substance called penicillinase, which destroyed the antibiotic. Less than ten years later, practically all the *S. aureus* bacteria had acquired this ability. The solution was to start using a synthetic form of penicillin, released in 1959, which penicillinase couldn't attack. It was called methicillin. But two years later, the first forms of *S. aureus* resistant to methicillin, namely the first MRSA, were being noticed.

The number of MRSA cases remained quite low until the 1980s. Although there were periodic outbreaks in hospitals, they could be kept under control by isolating patients. But MRSA gradually began to acquire resistance to other antibiotics, until they became the 'superbacteria' that they are today. At present, between 60 and 70 per cent of all the *S. aureus* found in hospitals are resistant to more than one antibiotic. A recent study reveals that, in Canada, 250,000 patients pick up a MRSA infection after being admitted to hospital and 8,000 of them die as a result. The number of infections has doubled in six years to reach a level of five out of every 1,000 people admitted. From the 1990s onwards, outbreaks of MRSA infections began to be detected outside health centres.

MRSA starts spreading

In December 2008, it was announced that MRSA and another resistant bacterium called VREF (*Enterococcus faecalis*, which is resistant to vancomycin) were being detected in several countries of South America, where 20 per cent of patients infected by MRSA died. Before 2005, there were no cases of MRSA recorded in the zone. It seems that the bacteria came from the United States.

In January 2009, it was found that MRSA had also infected swine herds in the Midwestern USA as well as swine workers. This demonstrated for the first time that the bacteria can pass from animals to humans. MRSA had been found in dogs, cats and horses, but no cases of this type of contagion in humans had been found. In Europe, Belgium, France, Italy and Spain are the countries where most resistant bacteria have been found in animals.

MRSA can still be treated with vancomycin, an antibiotic believed to the only one that's effective against superbacteria. In 2002, alarm bells started ringing when the first MRSA that were resistant to vancomycin were found in Michigan. Fortunately, only isolated cases were detected and, for some reason, it seems that the new resistance made them lose their original aggressiveness.

Resting on our laurels

As we have already seen, the best way to prevent resistances from being a problem is to keep producing new, more powerful drugs. This is what has happened so far. But the chain is in danger of breaking. Between 1930 and 1970, twelve new classes of antibiotics were developed. From 1970 until the beginning of this century, only two new ones appeared. The number of new antibiotics approved for human use has dropped from sixteen between 1983 and 1987 to five between 2003 and 2007. This means that there are fewer and fewer options. We relied too much on the antibiotics we had, and no one made sure that research continued at the necessary pace.

Let's see who wins ...		
Antibiotic	Year of first use	Year first resistance was detected
Streptomycin	1947	1947
Tetracycline	1952	1956
Methicillin	1959	1961
Gentamicin	1967	1970
Cefotaxime	1981	1983
Linezolid	2000	2001

Perhaps the error has been leaving the design of new antibiotics to the discretion of the pharmaceutical industry. The drug companies have ended up realizing that antibiotics aren't such a profitable product. There used to be as many as fifteen companies engaged in research into new antibiotics. Today, eight of them have left the field and two have considerably cut back their efforts, which means that the task has been left in the hands of only five companies (GSK, Novartis, AstraZeneca, Merck and Pfizer).

Antibiotics represent a business worth some $25,000 million per year. Nevertheless, the profits they bring in are much lower than those for other drugs – for example antidepressants or antihypertensives – since antibiotics are only taken for just over a week while the others are taken for years. Furthermore, the fact that resistances appear means that an antibiotic is useful for a decade at most, whereas the other drugs are effective more or less forever. And there's yet another paradox: the better an antibiotic is, the less doctors are advised to prescribe it, in order to prevent resistances from appearing. From the global health standpoint, it's better to keep it locked up in the safe for tough times that may come with the appearance of bacteria that can't be killed by anything else. From the company's point of view, however, this policy is hardly an incentive to design and market better drugs.

To all this must be added the extremely high cost of discovering new antibiotics. For example, GSK invested $70 million over seven years in genetic studies of new bacteria, trying to find common genes that could be targeted by new drugs. After all this effort, they only found five possible candidates, which are still being studied. Many more millions of dollars will be needed before it's known whether any of them can be used. In any other area, this kind of work would have come up with at least twenty potential drugs.

Hence, the economic imperative has given rise to a serious situation, as scientists have been warning for some time. If somebody doesn't take the lead and address the problem, the antibiotics we currently have will soon be obsolete. The disaster isn't going to happen tomorrow, but this isn't an impossible future. Hence, we need to find a solution now, while there's still time. Since we can't rely on the free market stimulus, it's been proposed that governments should invest more public money on antibiotics research. In recent years, the trend has begun to reverse and research into antibiotics is starting to revive, and it is to be hoped that this will slowly bear fruit once more.

The antibiotics of the future

Although one day we will manage to overcome the fragile situation we are now in, how long can we continue like this? Are the possibilities of designing new antibiotics never-ending, or will the time come when there will be no more new chemical combinations to test? The possibilities of generating new compounds are certainly not unlimited. But some people believe that we've only explored the tip of the iceberg. Most antibiotics come from substances generated by a relatively small group of microorganisms. Dr Eric Cundliffe of the University of Leicester, an expert on antibiotic resistance, says that we only need to pick up a handful of soil in order to have enough still unresearched microorganisms to obtain thousands of new substances with the potential for being useful antibiotics. If this really is the case, we needn't worry too much. We just need to keep investing time and money to discover the weapons that nature has given us for fighting our enemies.

There are other options too. One of the most promising methods of discovering new antibiotics works in a way that's opposite to what's been done so far. Instead of taking a natural or synthetic substance and looking at the effects it has on bacteria, an essential protein is chosen from a bacterium and attempts are then made to discover its structure. If we know the structure, we can theoretically design a specific chemical compound that will attach itself to the bacterium and inhibit it. Consequently, structural biochemistry, the field that studies the form of cell proteins, has recently become particularly relevant, not only in research for new antibiotics, but also for many other drugs. Using complex magnetic resonance imaging (MRI) or X-ray equipment, biochemists can deduce the appearance of most proteins. This information will then be passed on to a group of chemists who will design on paper the molecule that can best adapt to them and then synthesize it in the laboratory.

Recently, studies have been carried out in order to ascertain the possibility of using as antibiotics viruses called *bacteriophages*, which infect and kill bacteria. This may sound like a revolutionary concept, but a similar idea was first proposed more than 100 years ago. In Russia, a virus cocktail to combat bacterial infections had even been prescribed, but the practice was abandoned with the arrival of the first antibiotics. In 2006, use of the first virus-based treatment against *Listeria*, a bacterium that especially affects immunodeficient people and pregnant women, was approved in the United States and, more recently, we've seen applications of these bacteriophages in serious cases that didn't respond to antibiotics. Their use isn't yet general, but it's possible that, in future, such treatments will be increasingly important.

Antivirals

Just as antibiotics attack bacteria, so *antivirals* are drugs that allow us to thwart viruses. The main difference is that there aren't so many of them, and nor are they very effective, which is why viral infections are still much more difficult to treat. Furthermore, antivirals tend not to do away with the

> ## Myth and reality:
> ## low temperatures make us catch colds
>
> People say that if we don't wrap up well, we'll catch a cold. The illness even takes its name from the idea of being *cold*. Colds are caused by microbes and not by draughts. A scarf will be of little use if we inhale enough harmful viruses. No scientific experiment has yet managed to demonstrate that being cold increases the possibilities of falling ill because it makes us more susceptible to viruses or lowers our defences, even though some theories are being researched. The myth probably comes from the fact that it's true that colds are more frequent when temperatures are lower. But the reasons for this aren't yet totally clear.

microbe, since, in general, they only limit its growth. The best-known antivirals are those used to treat flu and AIDS. Other kinds are used to battle against herpes or hepatitis. Apart from these, not many others are available.

Antivirals are relatively recent drugs. Before they appeared, the only weapon against viral infections were vaccines. The first studies with antivirals date back to the 1960s, but it wasn't until the end of the twentieth century that most of those used today were discovered. In the last few decades, and thanks to advances that have enabled us to learn about virus genes, it's been possible to design more specific and effective antivirals. More than 100 are presently on the market.

Who pays the bills?

The cost of discovering, manufacturing, producing and distributing new drugs and vaccines is immense. Where does the money come from? Funding for defences against microbes comes from three main sources. First, different states invest part of their research budget for studying infectious diseases and their consequences. But government priorities don't always coincide with global interests. Moreover, the countries where the impact of infectious diseases is more serious tend to be those with the least resources to devote to research. Hence, rich countries need to make the effort to subsidize programmes that can be implemented in Africa, Asia and South America.

Second, a series of private foundations are responsible for a significant inflow of money in this field, thereby compensating for the lack of public funding. Perhaps the most important of all is the Bill & Melinda Gates Foundation, headed by the creator of Microsoft and his wife, with support from the billionaire Warren Buffett. Two of the world's richest people are giving a good part of their time and fortunes to covering fields of research that governments often put on hold. The Bill & Melinda Gates Foundation is the largest private organization of its kind in the world, and aims not only to improve healthcare around the globe, but also to reduce poverty and bolster education. The foundation began operations in 1994 and presently has a capital of about $35,000 million, with which it makes donations of some $1,500 million per year.

There are other organizations that bring together governments and private foundations with the idea of optimizing the use of resources and prioritizing goals. One of these is GAVI, The Vaccine Alliance, with headquarters in Switzerland, which is concerned with getting vaccines to places that need them most. It was founded in 2000 and, since then, has managed to vaccinate more than 213 million children, in a project that's believed to have saved more than 3 million lives. It presently has programmes underway

Revolutionary ideas

At the end of 2008, the Bill & Melinda Gates Foundation called on scientists to make proposals in highly specific areas of healthcare, especially AIDS, tuberculosis and malaria. Different ideas were wanted, new approaches to the usual problems were sought and the main difference from other mechanisms of financing was that it didn't require any kind of preliminary data demonstrating that the project was viable. The idea itself was enough.

One hundred million dollars were earmarked for the most impressive proposals, which included many that aimed to find effective vaccines against diseases that ravage developing countries. Each project chosen received an initial payment of $100,000, with the condition that, if the results were promising, a further million dollars would be donated. In the end, eighty-one projects were selected in the first round.

Examples of these risky ideas, which would be very unlikely to receive funding through normal channels, include the study of tomatoes as possible antivirals, a system using magnets to detect faeces of the malaria parasite in human blood, and a study on the effect that using laser before an injection might have on the effectiveness of a vaccine.

in more than seventy countries. GAVI members include the WHO, UNICEF, the World Bank, the Bill & Melinda Gates Foundation and representatives from the vaccine industry. GAVI launched a campaign to vaccinate all children by 2007 with the aim of obtaining funding from the private sector to pay for vaccines in poor countries and reduce the number of children, currently some 24 million, who were not being vaccinated against the commonest diseases.

The third essential element in the struggle against

infectious diseases consists of pharmaceutical companies. Not only do they spend a good portion of their budget on research with the aim of developing new drugs, but they also fund clinical trials, at least in part, and are responsible for producing enough doses of vaccines and drugs to guarantee that outbreaks can be contained. Without the ability of these corporations to produce drugs in large quantities and at great speeds, our defences against epidemics would be seriously weakened. It should also be borne in mind that investments of time and money that companies need to make to develop new drugs are very high indeed: around $1,000 million and a decade's research for each new product. And it's understandable that one of their priorities is to get their money back as fast as possible.

Then again, 'pharmaceutical companies have launched programmes to ensure that drugs are distributed to certain areas and these efforts are non-commercial', says Dr Arantxa Horga. 'In recent years, companies, governments, and NGOs have worked together much more, mainly because of public awareness and philanthropic efforts. Malaria, tuberculosis, and AIDS, are the diseases where there have been most benefits.' There are also ways of ensuring that the industry will cover some resource deficiencies that no one else can remedy. 'In the case of drugs for children,' Dr Horga says, 'which is a market that tends to be unprofitable for pharmaceutical companies, governments offer incentives for them to invest in research, for example by extending the period of their patents'[3] so that they can enjoy more time of exclusive benefits.

3   See footnote 2 on p. 70.

Shock troops

Under the auspices of the UN, the organization GOARN (Global Outbreak and Response Network) is responsible for sending teams of doctors and volunteers to zones where epidemics have been reported, in order to try to control them at source. Some members of these shock troops are from the WHO, and others are volunteers who often risk their lives without asking for any payment in return. There are also NGOs, like Doctors without Borders, that altruistically participate in these tasks.

Control and prevention

Apart from what we've seen so far, one of the most effective strategies for combating infections is to detect them in time and thereby prevent contagion. In this regard, agencies that monitor the appearance of epidemics and pandemics, at both local and global levels, are crucial. Swift action can prevent a great number of deaths, which means that governments must have plans to detect outbreaks of infectious diseases and then quickly inform the appropriate organizations so they can implement ways of isolating infected people and start preventive treatment for the noninfected population.

In the United States, the CDC (Centers for Disease Control and Prevention) is in charge of coordinating these kinds of responses, working with the WHO. With an annual budget of almost $9,000 million and employing 15,000 workers, it's the biggest government agency devoted to dealing with infections. Its main headquarters is in Atlanta and it has ten other centres in different parts of the country. Its equivalent in Europe is the ECDC (European Centre for Disease Prevention and Control), although some countries have their own centres – for example, the HPA (Health Protection Agency) in the United Kingdom and the InVS (Institut de veille sanitaire) in France.

One of the new tools for prevention is the Internet. By this means, it's possible to keep the world's population informed of the progress of an epidemic in real time. One example is the initiative called HealthMap (www.healthmap.org). This is a free website that reports on infections around the world, and governments and organizations like the WHO are constantly using its data. The information is obtained from all possible places, from press notes to official communiques by way of ProMED-Mail, a specialist discussion forum for professionals working in the field of infectious diseases. All the information from about 20,000 webpages is analysed every hour. Other websites containing similar initiatives include GPHIN (Global Public Health Intelligence Network), MEDISYS (Medical Information System), Argus and EpiSPIDER (Semantic Processing and Integration of Distributed Electronic Resources for Epidemiology).

4

The Danger of Knowing Too Much

Not all our problems relating to microorganisms are of natural origin. Humans can also cause outbreaks of infectious diseases, accidentally or intentionally. One example would be the use of microbes as weapons, a possibility that has always been very much in the forefront of the popular imaginary. This is a concept that seems generally to belong to the vocabulary of modern warfare, the dark side of recent scientific advances, but, in fact, this isn't so. The Romans, for instance, threw faeces at their enemies in the hope they would catch some disease, and besieging Mongol troops, affected by an epidemic, catapulted their dead inside the Caffa city walls. In the Middle Ages, animal or human corpses were used to contaminate water and spread the plague and, during the conquest of the West in America, colonists tried to infect Indians by giving them blankets used by smallpox patients. The use of insects is even older. It's believed that, in prehistoric times, bees and wasps were used in intertribal attacks.

During the Second World War, the Japanese army had a

plan to produce 5,000 million plague-infected fleas per year, to be showered on the allies, but didn't have time to see it through. However, the cruel experiments they carried out using biological weapons on prisoners of war in Unit 731 in Manchuria, under the command of Dr Shirō Ishii, are notorious.

Meanwhile, research in this area was also being carried out in the United States, and it's known that the departments of Defense and Agriculture were engaged in joint studies looking for microorganisms that the government might have deployed to its advantage in the war. In the Fort Detrick laboratories, the US army fermented almost 10,000 litres of anthrax in three large containers, as well as other microbes in smaller quantities. This was in violation of the 1925 Geneva Protocol which, only ratified by the US Senate in 1975, banned all kinds of chemical and biological warfare. Although the US Offensive Biological Weapons Program was officially renounced by President Nixon in 1968, sporadic research has still been carried out in the field since then.

On other occasions, viruses and bacteria have played an unforeseen part in wars, often in a way that benefited one or other party involved. It's calculated that two-thirds of the soldiers who died during the American Civil War were victims of malaria or yellow fever: 186,216 Union soldiers were killed by disease, 57,265 of whom died of dysentery. And let's recall once again that the conquest of Latin America was more a victory of microbes than of European armies.

Although, as far as we know, no one has recently used microscopic living beings to systematically attack soldiers or civilian populations, the danger is still present, now more than ever. The knowledge we have today, the relative ease with which the necessary materials can be obtained and the potentially devastating effects all mean that this is a particularly attractive weapon for some countries, and especially for terrorist groups, at least on paper. An American government report of 2005 titled *World at Risk* predicted that, in the next five years, it was highly likely that there would be at least one biological weapons attack somewhere in the world. Fortunately, the prediction was wrong.

The experts are pessimistic about the state of preparation for dealing with these weapons. The United States went from spending $271 million on biodefence at the end of the Clinton Administration to $4,000 million when George W. Bush was president, but it's believed that, if microbes were used in an attack on any city, the consequences would be devastating. In this chapter, I will discuss bioterrorism, but also the possibility of scientists causing epidemics as a result of errors made in the laboratory.

The paradox:
the more we research, the greater the danger

The fact that there's a possibility that armies or terrorists could use microorganisms only increases the risk of pandemics, not only because of the weapons themselves but also because of the dangers involved in the associated research. An infectious outbreak due to human action could be the result of a leak from a laboratory, which could cause a health crisis as serious as any premeditated biological attack. Most microorganisms susceptible to being used as biological weapons are relatively rare and don't tend to cause outbreaks or epidemics spontaneously. If it wasn't for their potential for misuse, some would be totally forgotten by now. However, if we are to protect ourselves against these threats, we must be able to carry out first-hand studies of the dangerous agents. But this would increase the likelihood of an accident in which the bacterium or virus being studied could be released unintentionally, or of ill-intentioned people gaining access to dangerous samples.

Deadly leak

It's happened at least once. The flu virus that caused the 1977 pandemic is believed to have escaped from a laboratory.

The virus of the H1N1 type that circulated in 1977 hadn't been seen in humans since 1957. When it reappeared, it was genetically identical to the type seen twenty years earlier. If the virus had been circulating in animal reservoirs, the easiest way of staying 'hidden' and beyond human control, it would have changed substantially because the flu virus evolves very quickly when it's free. The fact that it was the same as its predecessors would seem to suggest that the virus escaped from one of the laboratories where it was kept for study purposes.

One of the theories about the origin of the COVID-19 pandemic of 2020 was that the virus had escaped from a laboratory in Wuhan where the first outbreak occurred, though there is not yet any serious evidence to substantiate this claim.

One clear way out of this paradox is to find a way of being able to carry out research with proper guarantees of safety. It's necessary to make sure that none of the microorganisms will find a way to escape, accidentally or otherwise, and that the scientists who work with them are as protected to prevent contagion as they are monitored to ensure that they are not harbouring baneful ideas. Present-day security measures are purportedly so strict that errors are virtually impossible. Furthermore, the regulations are constantly being reviewed and improved. For example, at the beginning of 2009, the US government began to update laws related to the handling of biohazardous materials, in accordance with one of the executive orders signed by George W. Bush.

But things don't always work out as planned. In June 2009, it was announced that the US Army laboratory USAMRIID (United States Army Medical Research Institute of Infectious Diseases) in Maryland had 'found' 9,300 vials of 'unidentified' toxic organisms. They represented about 13 per cent of all the samples kept in the laboratory, which is the world leader in biological weapons research. In theory, each bacterium and each drop of blood must be perfectly labelled and inventoried to ensure that nobody can take them away without someone noticing. But, evidently, this wasn't the case. Some of the samples that appeared out of nowhere contained serum from soldiers who had died of viral haemorrhagic fever during the Korean War. Others contained Ebola, plague, anthrax and botulism. All of them had enormous toxic potential. It's believed that these were samples that researchers had forgotten to destroy when they left the laboratory, but this is no excuse for the poor security measures. Worst of all, there's no way of knowing whether any vials were lost or stolen, although the authorities say this is unlikely.

This shows that, for all the care taken when working with these kinds of dangerous materials, bureaucratic errors can result in some appearing and some disappearing without anybody being any the wiser, with the evident risk that this could be a temptation for bioterrorists. The US government insisted that new systems of inventorying samples should be introduced in order to avoid such blunders in future.

> ## Has anyone seen my virus?
>
> USAMRIID was caught up in another controversy in February 2009. A researcher found four vials of the Venezuelan equine encephalitis virus, which didn't appear in the database. Research in the centre immediately stopped until it was discovered where the mysterious vials had come from, and whether there were any more somewhere else.
>
> It's believed that someone had simply forgotten to enter the four vials in the list when the change was made from paper to electronic files in 2005.

Dangerous information

It's not only that samples of viruses and bacteria can fall into the wrong hands; the information about them is equally dangerous. In the struggle against biological agents, we need the information obtained in our studies to be freely distributed among other researchers around the world. However, certain articles normally published in scientific journals that are open to everyone could literally be used as 'recipes' for cultivating toxic microorganisms. Known as 'dual-use', this possibility has led to discussions about regulations concerning such studies and about which can be made public and which must remain secret. The problem, of course, is that the more that security measures are applied, and the more obstacles placed in the way of dissemination, the more slowly research in this area advances.

For example, as our genetic knowledge of viruses like that of the 1918 flu pandemic increases, public databases are being stocked with their genome sequences. If we know which pieces are needed to construct the most lethal virus that ever existed, what would stop a well-equipped terrorist group from reproducing it some day? According to Dr Martínez-Sobrido: 'Every day there are more possibilities of making aggressive viruses in a laboratory because there are more laboratories where this can be done, and the process is becoming fast and simple. The constraints are lessening all the time. Things that were once science fiction have now come true.'[4] Dr García-Sastre believes that the threat is more theoretical than real:

> There are faster and more efficient ways of making a biological weapon than reconstructing the 1918 flu virus. It's also a question of who gets there first. If terrorists ever manage to produce a deadly virus on the basis of our laboratory results, it's more than likely that we would have found a cure beforehand. Even with all the information we have, the many technical problems mean that this isn't an easy road for potential bioterrorists. It boils down to a very simple question of the balance between risks and benefits. The health benefits we gain from our research are thousands of times greater than the remote possibility that someone will misuse it.[5]

Anthrax

Among the group of microorganisms that can be used as weapons (see box on p. 98), one of the best known is anthrax. Otherwise known as *Bacillus anthracis*, anthrax is the only existing bacterium with a protective capsule made of

---

4   See footnote 1 on p. 27.
5   From an interview by the author with Adolfo García-Sastre [translation: JW].

Types of biological agents susceptible to being used as weapons (from more to less toxic, according to CDC in the United States)

Category A
Anthrax, smallpox, botulism, plague, tularaemia, and viral haemorrhagic fevers (like Marburg and Ebola)

Category B
Brucellosis, psittacosis, viral encephalitis, typhus, contamination of water reserves (cholera ...)

Category C
Tuberculosis, hantavirus ...

proteins. In fact, its name expresses confusion with the disease it causes, which, traditionally called carbuncle, gave rise to the Anglo-Saxon term anthrax. Derived from the Greek word for burning coal (ἄνθραξ), it refers to the skin lesions (carbuncles) characteristic of cutaneous anthrax infection.

Anthrax can be seen in people or animals and it presents different symptoms depending on where it enters the organism. If it comes via the respiratory tract, it initially shows flu-like symptoms that can lead to death from lung failure. If left untreated, it's fatal in more than 90 per cent of cases. Fortunately, antibiotics like penicillin have cut this figure to 45 per cent. If anthrax is ingested, for example by eating contaminated meat, it causes acute intestinal inflammation, which is fatal in 25–60 per cent of cases. The third, milder form is cutaneous, where only an ulcer appears at the point of entry. But, when not treated, it can be fatal in 20 per cent of these cases because, if the bacillus gets into the blood stream, it can cause a serious general condition.

Anthrax is a disease that's been known for millennia. In its cutaneous form, it's said to have been one of the ten plagues of Egypt described in the Bible. It's also mentioned in the *Iliad*. Usually it's only seen in people who work with animals because it's not transmitted between humans. The bacillus is able to form highly resistant structures called *spores* in which state it's protected and able to survive for decades as it awaits the ideal conditions to keep dividing. So, an infected cow or goat can release spores able to infect humans long after the animal's death. Nowadays, thanks to strict measures, there are few domestic animals with anthrax, but it had been a major problem until the end of the nineteenth century when Louis Pasteur discovered a vaccine that was effective against the bacillus that caused the disease.

A controversial name

Anthrax is the name of an American heavy metal band formed in 1981. During the 2001 anthrax attacks, the group decided to change its website. Entering www.anthrax.com in the browser took people straight to its page, which was confusing for those who wanted to know more about the disease and bioterrorism. The band decided to post useful health information and remove its musical content for a while.

In October 2001, the group announced in the press that it was considering changing to a more positive name. But, at a concert the following November, it declared that, despite all the bad vibes, there would be no change.

In terms of warfare, anthrax has the advantage of being very resistant and having a high mortality rate. Moreover, this microbe is relatively easy to obtain and handle. It's transmitted by air and tends not to spread beyond the target population. This is important for avoiding uncontrolled epidemics that could also affect those who are using it as a weapon. However, wind can scatter the spores widely and an attack could therefore cover a very large area. It's been calculated that, if a light aircraft, using a method similar to that employed for fumigating a field, dropped 100 kilos of anthrax on a city like Washington, it would cause 3 million deaths. If this happened at night, it would be difficult to detect and stop in time. It's also estimated that, if the bacteria were spread via the exhaust pipe of a Manhattan taxi, they could kill between 5 and 6 million people.

This quantity of spores is relatively small and could be within the reach of terrorists and nations that don't have a large army. In addition, in a laboratory, it would be quite easy to obtain anthrax that's resistant to penicillin and other antibiotics, which would enormously multiply the number of victims. This is why a possible attack is so greatly feared, and when it was suspected that Saddam Hussein was pursuing a biological weapons programme, not too many more excuses were needed for the United States to invade Iraq as a preventive measure.

As early as the nineteenth century, there was news of military use of anthrax. There was an attempt at mass production during the First World War, but it was abandoned in favour of mustard gas. During the Second World War, it was once again considered, and an especially aggressive version was even produced, but it was never used. The armies of both the United States and the United Kingdom have continued to carry out anthrax research ever since.

Bioterrorists in the USA

Just after the Twin Towers attack in New York on 11 September 2001, a case of bioterrorism crippled the United

States for months. An individual or group sent a total of seven letters containing anthrax spores to different addresses around the country. Twenty-two people were infected and five of them died. The first set of letters was sent from New Jersey on 18 September 2001, addressed to offices of national media outlets, among them NBC, CBS News and the *New York Post*. The recipients described the contents as a brownish powder. Two more letters with a higher dose of spores were sent from New Jersey on 9 October, this time to senators.

The handwritten notes accompanying the killer dust said, 'Death to America', 'Death to Israel' and 'Allah is great'. Everything suggested that the senders were Islamic extremists. The search for the culprits began at once and a reward of $2.5 million was offered to anyone who helped to find them. Immediately after the attacks, the FBI, under pressure from the White House, announced that this was a new round of attacks planned by Al Qaeda.

The situation was one of generalized panic. People were afraid that the next letter they opened would contain the killer dust. Post office employees were the most fearful of all, as they were handling thousands of envelopes and packages every day. But many of them didn't want to be vaccinated against the disease because they feared that the government would be using them as guinea pigs. The main reasons for their decision were lack of information and the conflicting views to which they were exposed. In the end, 10,000 postal service personnel received a two-month treatment with antibiotics.

In October, it was speculated that some military additives found in the spores were highly specific, which raised the suspicion that Iraq was responsible for the attack. Although several experts denied shortly afterwards that there was any additive, these data and others were used to justify the claim

The wrong man

Dr Steven Hatfill, virologist and expert in biological weapons, was named a 'person of interest' by the US Department of Justice in the case of the anthrax terrorist attacks. The FBI searched his home and the media reported the news.

It all began because, in 1999, after several threats of attacks using anthrax hidden in letters, which turned out to be fake, Hatfill had been asked to write a report about the likelihood of such a terrorist act. It's not clear who commissioned the report. Some sources say it was the CIA; others conclude that it was an initiative of Hatfill and his colleagues.

In the end, it turned out that Hatfill had nothing to do with bioterrorism. Not long afterwards, he sued the US government for damages, saying it had 'destroyed his reputation'. He was paid $5.8 million in compensation.

It was proven, however, that Hatfill was indeed guilty of something: forging his PhD certificate.

that Iraq had weapons of mass destruction and that swift action was needed to avoid more serious attacks.

It wasn't until May 2002 that investigators began to link the anthrax with laboratories in the United States. To general surprise, analysis of the spores showed that, in all cases, they came from the strain called Ames, which had been studied first at USAMRIID and then distributed to some twenty laboratories around the world. Owing to its dangerous nature, only a very limited number of people had access to it. In theory, this should have made it easier to find the perpetrator. But the investigations dragged on for several years, apparently without any conclusions being reached. Then, on 29 July 2008, Bruce Ivins, a 62-year-old scientist, committed suicide with an overdose of analgesics, after which it was publicly announced that, following an investigation of almost seven years, the FBI was about to name him as the culprit.

The use of new genetic techniques that had appeared in the previous few years had at last enabled scientists to study the variants of the Ames strain that were distributed around the different laboratories. They had fully sequenced between ten and twenty bacteria genomes. There were more than 1,000 samples distributed around the world but only eight genetically matched the ones in the letters. And all of them came from the consignment called RMR-1029. This was kept at USAMRIID and Bruce Ivins had had exclusive responsibility for it since it was first cultivated and studied in 1997. It also happened that, immediately prior to the attacks, Ivins had spent more time than usual in the building where RMR-1029 was kept, often outside working hours. Furthermore, when the FBI started to investigate, Ivins gave them the wrong samples in order to mislead them.

It is believed that Ivins had had psychological problems since at least 2000. In 2002 the FBI, searching for information, asked the American Society for Microbiology to turn over its list of 43,000 members, and it ended up thoroughly scrutinizing sixty of the country's leading anthrax experts in relation with the case. The microbiologist Nancy Haigwood had suggested that they should check out Ivins, stating that his deranged behaviour had been making her life impossible for twenty years. The FBI asked Haigwood to meet Ivins wearing a wire, to see if she could extract information. Although she initially agreed, she later backed out because she was scared. In any case, this was most probably the beginning of the end for Ivins.

If Ivins was solely responsible, his motives aren't known and neither was it ascertained how he managed to make the anthrax easy to inhale, a process that required military knowledge (see box opposite). Moreover, some reports say that between ten and a hundred people had had access to the vials of anthrax in Ivins's keeping. One of the weak points of the theory is that the FBI hasn't been able to reproduce the exact format in which the spores in the letters were found, which would mean that things aren't as simple as they appear and that, consequently, Ivins would never have been able to produce them by himself in a few surreptitious night-time sessions in the laboratory.

The FBI asked the scientific community of experts from the US National Academy of Sciences to analyse the data independently and confirm that the experimental methods it had used were appropriate and its conclusions correct. A committee of fifteen experts finally began this investigation at the end of July 2009 but didn't manage to shed any light on the matter. Perhaps we will never know for sure whether Ivins was the anthrax killer and, if he was, whether he acted alone or in concert with others.

The return of smallpox?

Smallpox is another disease that tends to be mentioned when people talk about bioterrorism. As I said above, it's been eradicated from the planet, but the virus still exists. Two samples are being kept, protected with elaborate security measures, one in the United States (in the CDC headquarters in Atlanta) and the other in Russia (first in the Moscow Research Institute of Viral Preparations and, later, in Siberia). Keeping them was a controversial decision at the time because of the potential danger the samples represented, but it's believed to be important to have samples available in case the virus needs to be studied. Once again, it's thought that the benefits outweigh the risks. The plan

The silicon mystery

One of the keys to the Ivins case is whether or not the spores were manipulated to make them more dangerous (or, as the experts say, to give them 'weapon quality'). If this were the case, the chances that a microbiologist like Ivins could have done this alone are very slim.

At first it was said that, yes, the spores had been treated to make them more volatile. Later, the experts discarded this verdict. One of the ways of preventing spores from clumping together, and to ensure that they can spread more easily, is to cover them with a layer of silicon. And, in fact, silicon traces were detected in the samples. It was believed at first that this was proof of manipulation, but it was later decided that the silicon had become incorporated in the spores naturally and not with express intention in a laboratory.

It's still not clear what kinds of manipulation the bacillus underwent. Some FBI reports say that the spores contain neither silicon nor any other additive.

was to destroy them at the end of the twentieth century, but then it was decided to give them an indefinite reprieve. With the hypothetical possibility that smallpox could be used as a bioterrorist weapon, research programmes have been reactivated with the aim of finding safer and more effective vaccines and treatments.

But we can't be totally sure that the two samples of the virus are the only ones in existence, especially after the collapse of the Soviet Union and all the problems arising from that. There are rumours claiming that the Russian army was working with the smallpox virus in the 1980s, trying to create a hybrid with the even more lethal Ebola virus. This means that there might be samples of the former in more than one Russian laboratory. Someone could have managed to get hold of a small amount and that would be sufficient to create a problem: the virus is simple to cultivate, is stable for a long time and spreads very easily through the air. It therefore has the ideal qualities for use as a biological weapon. Given this possibility, any precaution is paltry.

5

Forgotten Diseases and New Diseases

In this chapter and the next, I will talk about some of the most important currently seen infectious diseases (apart from the four great modern epidemics, described in Part II). By this I mean those that have, for years, been causing the greatest health and social problems. Some are newcomers, like COVID-19. Others belong to the group of 'forgotten diseases', or infections that have coexisted with us for some time but that, due to the fact that they mainly tend to affect the poorest countries, don't receive the attention they deserve. Some are more deadly than others. Some respond to treatment and some don't. Whatever the case, it's important to bear in mind that they exist, that they have a significant impact and, although they are not always front-page news, we could all fall victim to them some day.

The new infectious diseases

These are some of the infectious diseases that have appeared most recently, together with the year in which they were discovered:

Ebola (1976)
Legionella (1977)
Lyme disease (1982)
AIDS (1983)
SARS (2002)
MERS (2012)
COVID-19 (2019)

Meningitis

Meningitis is an inflammation of the membranes covering the brain. It's relatively infrequent in the northern hemisphere, although there have been a few sporadic outbreaks. However, it's a very serious problem in some African countries, especially in the zone stretching from Ethiopia to Senegal. It can be caused by different kinds of microbes, but one of the most serious forms is that due to *Neisseria meningitidis*, also known as meningococcus, which is transmitted by saliva. If untreated, it kills 50 per cent of those infected. Even with antibiotics, 10 per cent die and another 25 per cent can suffer serious sequelae. There's an outbreak of meningitis every year, starting in January or February, and disappearing after three or four months with the first rains, usually after May. The reasons for this annual cycle are still unknown. Despite having the advantage of precise knowledge about the season in which cases of meningitis will appear in Africa, it's not yet possible to predict where they will appear, or how serious the year's outbreak is going to be.

In 2009, a particularly intense meningitis epidemic hit the area covering Nigeria, Burkina Faso, Mali and Niger, with more than 25,000 possible cases of infection and 1,500 dead (although confirmed figures are 13,500 infected and 930 dead). It began earlier than previous years and was the worst outbreak since 1996 when, in a similar epidemic, 250,000 people were infected and 25,000 died. That time it affected ten different countries.

The vaccines used must cover several bacteria. The meningococcus vaccine hasn't been improved since the 1960s and only gives protection for a short period (about three years). Work is being done to produce a better and cheaper vaccine than the one we have now. However, the vaccine against *Haemophilus influenzae* type B (Hib), another of the bacteria that causes the disease, is effective and has managed to curb this kind of meningitis ever since it has been given in many countries as part of the children's vaccination programme. But the number of doses arriving in the stricken zones is often insufficient to cover the whole population at risk. Getting the vaccine distributed fast enough and everywhere it's needed is one of the main obstacles to controlling the disease.

Cholera

Millions of people around the world live in zones where they are at risk of contracting cholera. There are usually more than 100,000 victims of this disease every year. Normally, it's transmitted in drinking water contaminated by faeces of infected people, so general health and hygiene conditions, especially filtering and chlorinating water, have a huge influence on the evolution of the disease, which is why it's presently only seen in developing countries. The last cholera pandemic was in the 1970s but, since then, there have been outbreaks with a certain frequency. For reasons that are as yet unknown, cholera epidemics also follow seasonal patterns.

The main symptom of cholera is the sudden onset of severe watery diarrhoea brought on by the toxin secreted by *Vibrio cholera*, the bacterium responsible for the disease. In 5 per cent of cases, unless treated urgently, it kills within a few hours of the symptoms appearing. Although antibiotics help, the most important thing is intensive rehydration to prevent shock.

Infected people who don't die acquire immunity against future infection. It was thought that it lasted for some years, but recent studies suggest that it may only give protection for a few months in some cases. One obstacle to eradicating cholera is asymptomatic infection. This occurs 250 times more frequently than it does with symptoms, which means that many people can transmit the disease without having the faintest idea that they are infected.

There are three standard oral vaccines against cholera: Dukoral, Shanchol and Euvichol. The highly effective and relatively cheap Dukoral, costing between five and nine euros per vaccine, is the most commonly used of the three. Like the other two, it's administered orally, but the problem is that it has to be kept cold, and two doses must be taken with at least a week between them. Outside the big cities, these are very difficult conditions to achieve in many parts of Africa, which is why the WHO doesn't believe it's viable to support mass vaccination strategies. Vaxchora is another orally administered vaccine that has recently come to the fore.

At the end of 2008, as a cholera epidemic ravaged Zimbabwe, with thousands of dead and tens of thousands sick, the government of the dictator Robert Mugabe tried to play down the figures and denied that there was any problem. Witnesses say that the roads were covered with filth and refuse, with maggots and flies proliferating very near the houses. In hospitals – with no electricity or running water, and sometimes without even doctors or nurses, since many of them had left the country (up to 50 per cent after 2000) – sick people were crammed together, making it easier for the infection to spread among them. Owing to the country's political problems, bodies accumulated without time to bury them, decomposing and further contaminating drinking water sources.

Zimbabwe had had one of Africa's best health systems, including an important research centre at the University of Zimbabwe, but all of that had been lost in the preceding years because of political instability. It had been decades since the country had had a cholera outbreak except for a few isolated cases that were normally dealt with within a few weeks. It was impossible to calculate the extent of this new epidemic or when it might be curbed. It spread through neighbouring countries in southern Africa, including South Africa, Zambia, Mozambique and Congo. Other serious cholera outbreaks in Africa include that in Angola in 2006–7 (85,000 cases, with 5 per cent dead) and in South Africa in 2002 (116,000 cases, and 1 per cent dead).

Since 2010 there have been a dozen cholera epidemics around the world. The most serious of these were in Yemen (beginning in 2017 and still ravaging that war-torn country, with more than 0.5 million cases) and Haiti/Dominican Republic (with some 900,000 people infected and nearly 10,000 dead).

Cinematographic viruses

The film *Outbreak*, starring Dustin Hoffman as a USAMRIID coronel who has to stop an outbreak of haemorrhagic fever in an American town, was premiered in 1995. The virus responsible for this is called Motaba in the film but, in fact, it's identical to Ebola. The epidemic begins thanks to an infected monkey in a case resembling the first known outbreak of another haemorrhagic fever, namely that which happened in Marburg, Germany. Coincidentally, the film was premiered some months after an Ebola outbreak in Zaire. This led to general debate about the real possibility of a similar situation in the United States and the plans that the CDC might have to contain it.

Similar viruses star in the zombie films *28 Days Later* (2002) and *28 Weeks Later* (2007). The epidemics begin in a similar way, with infected monkeys. This time, besides the haemorrhagic fever, the disease causes an aggressive state of rage in the victims, who then violently attack everyone.

Contagion (2011) is one of the films that most realistically shows the effects of a pandemic. It takes SARS as a model, but the virus that causes this fictional disease is much more aggressive. The film gained popularity during the COVID-19 outbreak because it resembled what was actually happening.

The Andromeda Strain (1969), a novel by Michael Crichton, which was made into a film in 1971, is about a virus that arrives from space and threatens to cause an uncontrollable outbreak. Some virologists quote the title of the film today when they want to refer to a possible outbreak of an unknown virus that we'd be unable to curb.

An earlier example of epidemic control in cinema is *Panic in the Streets*, a film from 1950 in which Richard Widmark has to stop a criminal who is infected with a pulmonary form of plague before he spreads it throughout the city of New Orleans.

West Nile virus

Until the end of the twentieth century, few people in the developed countries had heard about West Nile virus (also known as WNV). It mainly affects birds, but can spread to humans by way of mosquito bites. While 20 per cent of cases present headaches, aches and pains, and inflamed lymph nodes, all of which disappear in a few weeks, 80 per cent are asymptomatic. Relatively infrequent and limited to tropical regions in particular, the disease was described for the first time in 1937, in Uganda, although it's speculated that the virus had been around for quite some time. Some people even suggest that Alexander the Great was the first renowned victim, while others believe he died of malaria or typhoid fever.

The virus became famous when it first entered America in 1999, via New York. It's believed that it came with a mosquito travelling on a plane coming from Africa. There was considerable alarm in the city. One of the first signs that something was happening was the death of a large number of birds in the Bronx Zoo, together with a series of cases of an unidentified illness in humans, which started affecting the neighbourhood of Queens. In the first summer, there were sixty-two serious cases and seven deaths in the city. After that, the virus started spreading outwards to reach the West coast of the United States in 2002. From the onset of the epidemic until 2004, there were 16,000 cases and 660 deaths. By 2007, some 3,600 people throughout the country were very ill with the infection and nearly 125 had died, a fatality rate of below 4 per cent.

There is no treatment or vaccine for the disease, so the most effective strategy is to focus on transmission. The New York City authorities tried to halt the initial outbreak by spraying Central Park with large doses of insecticides, delivered by tanker trucks on summer nights. People were also advised not to walk in the park after sunset, when the mosquitoes were starting to appear. For the moment, outbreaks in Europe have been sporadic and minor; 209 cases were reported in the summer of 2020, for example, with 21 deaths in Greece and Spain.

Ebola

The Ebola virus causes haemorrhagic fever with heavy bleeding, which is often fatal. It belongs to one of the five families of viruses – among them Marburg and Lassa fever – which cause similar symptoms. From the time Ebola was discovered in 1976 through to the beginning of this century, only about 1,000 people had died, mainly in Central Africa, so this disease was a rarity. But Ebola has acquired unexpected prominence because of two big recent outbreaks, also in Africa. One, lasting from 2013 to 2016, killed more than 11,000 people (the largest number so far), while a smaller outbreak with a death toll of 2,280 began in Congo in 2018 and was officially declared over at the end of June 2020. The 2013 epidemic is important not only because of its magnitude, but also it was the first to affect countries outside Africa. The United Kingdom, Italy, Spain and the United States recorded Ebola victims for the first time. They had all become infected in Africa but none of them led to the start of an outbreak in their countries of origin.

The 2018 outbreak was the second most lethal ever recorded (with an average mortality of 66 per cent) and the first in which experimental antiviral drugs and a vaccine were given. The vaccine had been developed by Merck during the previous epidemic and was finally available to be administered to more than 300,000 people during this latest outbreak. Preliminary data suggests that it not only gave 80 per cent protection, but it reduced the severity of the disease in those who were affected. Furthermore, two new drugs, mAB114 and REGN-EB3, both based on antibodies that block the virus, were initially tested and were found to significantly reduce the number of deaths. They were therefore immediately given to as many patients as possible. Although these drugs and the vaccine could change the future prospects of Ebola, which was previously untreatable, the mortality rate of the disease is still quite high despite this progress.

There are six known types of the Ebola virus: Zaire, Sudan, Taï Forest (formerly called Côte d'Ivoire), Bundibugyo, Reston and, the most recent addition, Bombali (first reported in 2018). Infection by three of these variants (Zaire, Sudan and Bundibugyo) are fatal in 25–90 per cent of cases, mainly depending on the quality of the treatment received by those affected. The only course of action is to treat the symptoms that appear. Humans are normally infected by contact with sick animals, especially monkeys, so Ebola is a problem of nonurban zones, and mostly in African countries. In 2005, Ebola epidemics in Gabon and Congo were believed to have been caused by infected bats.

In 2008, a variant of the Ebola virus, called Reston, was identified in pigs in the Philippines. It was the first case of Ebola being detected in an animal that wasn't a primate. As with humans, the pigs might have been infected by bat droppings that had fallen into their food. This type of virus had been observed for the first time in 1989 in Reston, Virginia, among a group of monkeys that, still in quarantine, were to be used for research purposes. The monkeys came from the Philippines and it was found that people who'd had contact with them had antibodies against the virus, although only one of them had developed symptoms similar to those of flu.

There were outbreaks of the Reston virus among humans in the Philippines between 1992 and 1996, but nobody died of the disease.

Being infected by a macaque is unusual. However, there are many more people who have contact with pigs, which is why the discovery of the Reston virus in these animals could pose a significant danger for humans. The virus is destroyed by heat, so eating pork presents no risk as long as it's well cooked. It's believed that some Ebola epidemics in Africa have been preceded by unusual spikes in pig deaths, which suggests that they've transmitted the virus to humans. The virus hadn't infected any human working with pigs until January 2009, when a farmer tested positive for antibodies against it. In February that year, four more cases were discovered. None of the infected people presented serious symptoms. The Reston virus hasn't yet caused any fatalities, so it would need to become more aggressive if it were to set off any serious epidemic. This is precisely what can happen if one virus exchanges information with another. And it often occurs when more than one virus infects the same pig.

Haemorrhagic fevers like Ebola are the worst of all known such diseases because they are so aggressive. Fortunately, this also limits their reach, as patients are usually quickly detected and isolated before large-scale epidemics ensue. However, from time to time, an outbreak gets out of control and can spread to neighbouring countries, as we've recently seen. Nevertheless, the chances of their causing a pandemic are, in principle, low because of the characteristics I've described.

In any case, we shouldn't make the mistake of believing that Ebola and related diseases are just a problem for Africa. The great ease of travelling nowadays means that an outbreak can swiftly move to other countries, as we've seen with some cases of Ebola this century. Moreover, there exist other risk situations that are particular to developed countries. For example, in March 2009, a researcher in the Bernhard Nocht Institute of Tropical Medicine in Hamburg, Germany, was accidentally exposed to Zaire Ebola, one of the more toxic variants of the virus, after pricking herself with a contaminated needle. Although she was wearing the proper protection typical of laboratories where Ebola is studied, the needle punctured her skin.

Needlestick injuries usually aren't fatal since few viruses get into the bloodstream this way. A similar case happened in 2004 at USAMRIID, and the scientist was saved without requiring treatment, possibly because he wasn't infected by any virus. In the German case, they weren't taking any chances. The researcher was immediately isolated and, in less than 48 hours, she was given an experimental vaccine which, produced in Canada, had never been tried with humans, although it had proven effective with monkeys. In the end, she didn't develop the disease, but no one can claim that the vaccine protected her because it isn't known if the virus from the needle got into her bloodstream. After three weeks, the maximum incubation time known for Ebola, she was released from hospital, although she remained on sick leave because the situation had been so stressful.

Dr Luis Martínez-Sobrido recalls:

When a virus infects someone, it normally does so in very low quantities. In a laboratory, however, work is done with much higher concentrations in order to store and study the viruses well. So, the risk of infection is much higher than it is among the normal population. Nowadays, we have better knowledge of viruses, how they are transmitted, the diseases they cause, what protections are needed, and the restrictions and controls for working with them are much stricter than they were a few years ago. It's also possible to eliminate the parts of a virus known to make it more toxic, as occurs when

Types of microbiology laboratories

Depending on the degree of safety measures, there are four kinds of laboratories engaged in research on microorganisms.

Level 1: work is done with organisms that don't cause diseases or that represent the smallest risk for health. Low-level precautions are taken.

Level 2: microbes causing diseases but that aren't easily transmitted by air in the laboratory can be studied (for example, HIV and salmonella). Staff must be trained, access to the laboratory is restricted, and biocontainment systems are used to ensure that the microbes don't spread.

Level 3: the microbes studied cause serious diseases or death if inhaled (for example, anthrax or SARS). Safety measures are stricter, and the laboratory air is filtered.

Level 4: serious diseases transmitted through air and against which there is no vaccine or treatment are studied (for example, Ebola). The laboratories are sealed, and researchers work in ventilated diving suits. They must also go through decontamination showers and ultraviolet light chambers. This type is unusual.

vaccines are made, so that we can feel more relaxed about working with them.[6]

Marburg: the other serious haemorrhagic fever

Marburg fever, caused by a virus whose effects aren't unlike those of Ebola, was first identified in 1967. It originated

6   See footnote 1 on p. 27.

in Africa but was discovered in Germany (in the town of Marburg and others) and the former Yugoslavia when there was an outbreak that affected thirty-one people, seven of whom died. The outbreak began among scientists in laboratories who were working with monkeys imported from Uganda. Some of the animals had died for unknown reasons, but it didn't occur to anyone that the disease could be transmitted to humans by contact with monkey fluids. The infection started with flu-like symptoms which, within twenty-four hours, had worsened to include diarrhoea and vomiting blood. As with Ebola, there's no treatment, and vaccines that seem to work with monkeys are being studied.

Marburg affects primates, although it's thought that bats could act as a reservoir, thus concealing the virus between one outbreak and the next. The mortality rate is very high, between 20 and 100 per cent, but it has only caused some 500 fatalities since it was discovered. Of the 374 people infected in the 2005 outbreak in Angola, 329 died (almost 88 per cent). Between 1998 and 2000, 128 people died in Congo, most of

The cure is worse than the disease

In Africa, epidemics like Ebola or Marburg can be made worse by hospitals. These are such deadly diseases that they often kill the infected person before there's time to infect anyone else because, in rural areas, the population density is very low. The fact of taking an infected person to hospital in the city means more possibilities for contact with other people, thus making contagion easier if there are no strict control measures. Another contributing factor is poor sanitary conditions in these hospitals where, for example, it's common practice to reuse needles because there aren't enough. It isn't unusual for someone who is admitted with malaria (which is curable) to catch Ebola and die from it.

them miners. It's suspected that this was because they came into contact with sick bats living in the mines.

The 'forgotten' diseases

A number of diseases have been labelled as forgotten (see box) because it seems that, in the West, it's a case of out of sight, out of mind, despite the harm they still cause in certain countries. These diseases are not at all rare. Some are more common than others, but it's calculated that, taken together, they affect 1,400 million people around the world. Notable among them are two major infections, Chagas disease and dengue, which I will discuss separately.

'Forgotten diseases' covered by the WHO programme
Chagas disease
Dengue
Buruli ulcer
Dracunculiasis
Fasciolosis
Trypanosomiasis
Leishmaniasis
Leprosy
Lymphatic filariasis (elephantiasis)
Zoonotic diseases (transmitted by animals)
Onchocerciasis
Helminthiasis
Snakebite
Trachoma
Bouba (frambesia tropica or yaws)

By way of proof of the scant interest in these diseases, one could cite the fact that 80 per cent of the $2,700 million invested in researching new cures for health problems affecting developing countries are allocated for studying AIDS, tuberculosis and malaria. The other 20 per cent has to be divided among all the rest. Between 1975 and 2004, only 21 out of a total of 1,556 drugs approved for use with humans were for treating the forgotten diseases. About 70 per cent of the research for this group of diseases was paid for by governments (42 per cent by the United States). Proportionally speaking, Ireland and the United States are the countries that give the most (about $4 per capita). Since 2007, the United States government has promised $470 million for this initiative, and the United Kingdom a further $75 million. In addition, 21 per cent of funding comes from NGOs, most of it from the Bill & Melinda Gates Foundation (18 per cent, or $34 million).

The Bill & Melinda Gates Foundation has experience in this field. In 2000 it began with a donation of $20 million for a programme to eliminate lymphatic filariasis, which causes the disease known as elephantiasis in which the skin thickens and the extremities or scrotum can swell to enormous proportions. The source is microscopic worms transmitted by mosquito bites. At the start of the programme, the drugs for treating elephantiasis only reached 25 million people distributed among twelve different countries. By 2009 they were available for 570 million people in forty-eight countries.

The most tragic thing is that many of these diseases can be prevented and treated by drugs that cost no more than 50 cents per person per year. One of the keys to reducing the impact of the forgotten diseases is to get the big drug companies to donate millions of treatments to the people who need them. Merck, GSK, Pfizer, Johnson & Johnson and MedPharma have all pledged to participate in a programme of free distribution of drugs against these diseases. I will speak briefly about some of the more relevant among them below.

Chagas disease

Chagas disease is found in the most impoverished zones of Latin America. It's the region's most worrying parasitic ailment and the main cause of heart problems. It's believed that about 18 million people are infected, with about 43,000 deaths every year. In countries like Bolivia, up to 20 per cent of the population could be affected by Chagas disease, which is the fourth main cause of death in the country. It's chronic and asymptomatic in 60 per cent of those affected, but it can cause serious heart disorders in 30 per cent. The WHO has recently revived the programme against Chagas disease after cancelling it some time ago when it was believed that the infection had been beaten.

The Brazilian doctor Carlos Chagas accidentally discovered the disease that now bears his name a century ago. He was working in an antimalaria campaign in Brazil when he realized that an unusual parasite was showing up in some blood samples. It was *Trypanosoma cruzi*. Chagas gave it this name in honour of his mentor Oswaldo Cruz. The cause of the infection is the 'barber bug', or *vinchuca* (technical name *Triatoma infestans*), an insect that lives in the cracks of houses or thatched roofs of rural huts and bites mainly at night. Chagas was able to describe the microbe, the insect that transmits it and the symptoms of the disease – a rare feat in the study of infections.

Treatments against Chagas disease are only effective in under-15-year-olds, and in adults who have it in the early stages. For more than thirty years, benznidazole and nifurtimox, which have numerous side effects, have been used, and it has found that, although they don't cure the disease, they do prevent heart complications in adults. No better alternatives have been discovered yet, mainly because of a lack of research in the field.

Chagas disease is found around the world today, mainly amongst immigrants from endemic zones. Hence, it's important that doctors should know how to recognize it. In Southern Europe, there has been a recent increase in the number of infected people, many of whom have immigrated from countries like Bolivia, and rigorous medical check-ups have been set up to detect whether the disease has pro-gressed to the symptomatic phase. In some cultures, it's still assumed that Chagas disease is fatal because only the serious, incurable cases were previously visible. In Europe, in order to educate the population and ensure that the maximum number of people receive treatment, organizations like Spain's ASAPECHA (Association of Friends of People with Chagas Disease) have been established to inform people suf-fering from the disease and their families, and to help them cope with it.

Dengue

Dengue is the insect-borne disease that has proliferated most in the world this century. It is mainly present in the tropics and is eminently urban because the *Aedes aegypti*, the mos-quito that transmits the virus that causes it, prefers to live in cities where it easily reproduces in pools of water. It is calculated that tens of millions of people are infected in the tropics. Two-fifths of the world's population are in areas of risk. More and more cases are being seen, spurred mainly by migration from the country to cities. Some studies calculate that there are between 50 and 100 million new cases every year. The WHO has identified at least 100 countries where it's endemic. In Thailand, for example, 83 out of every 100,000 people get dengue on a year-by-year basis.

Normally, the symptoms include a high temperature with severe muscular and joint pains – the so-called dengue fever – but it's not fatal. In a small proportion of cases, however, it presents as haemorrhagic fever with significant bleeding that can cause the patient to die. It's still not known why this more serious form of the disease appears. One of the theories is that it happens when a person is infected with the virus for a second time, but only with a long enough period between the mosquito bites. If the second bite follows closely on the first, possibly because there are many mosquitoes in the zone, the person will probably still have enough immunity to check the virus. If they are more spaced out, the second bite can be fatal. So, trying to stop dengue by killing mosquitoes can have the opposite effect to what's desired. Unless they are all eliminated, the bites will be further apart in time and the number of serious cases would therefore increase.

Possible vaccines are being researched, but none is yet ready for use. Neither is there any effective treatment. For the time being, the best defence against the disease is protection using mosquito nets and insecticides. In 2009, the results of a study carried out in the Amazon were published. In this research, the mosquitoes used had been modified in the laboratory so they would pass on a toxic substance to their larvae. In other words, the adult mosquitoes themselves delivered the 'insecticide' to their offspring. The first results showed a big drop in the number of mosquitoes in the zone, thanks to this new technique.

Dengue had been eliminated from South America by the mid-twentieth century but, in the early years of the twenty-first century, it's making a strong comeback and we still don't know much about the causes. It's speculated that climate change (see box), fast urbanization, and discontinuation of use of insecticides might have had some influence. The outbreaks tend to appear in the rainy season, coinciding, too, with the famous Brazilian carnivals, which means that a large number of tourists could catch the disease. In Rio de Janeiro, there have been cases in the affluent neighbourhoods, and even some deaths. A tourist coming from South America or Southeast Asia who presents with fever might have contracted dengue, although this isn't the first disease doctors think of, which can delay the diagnosis.

An additional danger of global warming

It's believed that global warming can contribute to the increased incidence of many infectious diseases, since it's expanding the zones where the insects transmitting them can live. The first theories about this possibility date back to the end of the twentieth century. Some people believe they are exaggerated, since it's not only temperature that influences the fact that a mosquito can live in a geographic zone and transmit diseases therein. In some cases, for example, an animal that can act as a reservoir is necessary. Other experts agree that these obstacles do exist, but believe that, since there's been no exposure to these diseases in the new areas where viruses are spreading, the basic immunity would be lower, and the initial death toll could be very high.

Dengue is becoming a serious problem in the southernmost part of South America as well, especially in Argentina and Bolivia. Recently, there have been between 10,000 and 30,000 cases in Argentina and, in Bolivia, up to 114,000. On 9 April 2009, the authorities confirmed that there had been

150 cases of infection in Buenos Aires. Most of them weren't fatal, although the first cases presenting with serious haemorrhagic fever have now been recorded.

The chances of an epidemic of dengue outside the areas where it's endemic are low, but it's not impossible. The tiger mosquito (*Aedes albopictus*), which has settled in the Iberian Peninsula and other areas of the south of Europe in recent years, belongs to the same family as the dengue-transmitting mosquito, but it's less efficient. Socioenvironmental determinants, however, mean that a possible epidemic in the Mediterranean region would probably be small and manageable.

Hand, foot and mouth disease

A viral disease mainly affecting young children – hand, foot and mouth disease (HFMD) – shouldn't be confused with aphthous fever, or foot-and-mouth disease, which is found among animals and entails significant economic loss to farmers if not dealt with in time. The symptoms of the human disease are mild, usually mouth ulcers and fever but, in a small percentage of cases, it can affect the brain and cause death. The sequelae it leaves are also serious because it can attack nerves. Contagion occurs through contact with saliva, mucous and faeces. At present there's no treatment and no vaccine ready for use.

There have been major outbreaks, especially in Asia. In 1997 in Malaysia, 2,600 cases of the disease were detected, and 29 people died. In 1998, the numbers rose sharply to 129,000 cases with 78 dead. In 2008, some 500,000 people were infected with the virus in China, and 200 of them died. An unusual outbreak was again detected in China in 2009. The cause of the outbreaks was the so-called enterovirus 71, one of several viruses that can induce the disease, and also one of the kinds that most affect the brain, leading to a fatal infection.

Little is known about enterovirus 71, and it is also unknown whether it could ever come to spread around the globe. Like the flu virus, it has considerable ability to mutate. This means that, in theory, there could be a major pandemic of hand, foot and mouth disease if the virus was capable of spreading fast. The experts disagree about the level of concern enterovirus 71 deserves. Some believe that it could come to be a serious problem, while others doubt that it would ever go beyond local outbreaks of low virulence. Everyone agrees, though, that it's necessary to keep monitoring and studying cases of the disease in order to learn more about the virus and thus be able to predict the seriousness and extent of outbreaks.

6

Coronaviruses and Future Pandemics

Coronaviruses: the new plague?

At the beginning of this century, a new family of viruses dramatically joined the list of the most dangerous microbes: the coronaviruses. In fact, coronaviruses have been known since the 1960s: they cause common colds and also infect animals. They were named thus in 1968 when the electronic microscope showed that they have a structure with a series of protrusions on the surface, reminding scientists of the sun's corona (though it also resembles a king's crown, the image most associated with these viruses today). They are larger than the viruses that typically cause infections (125 nanometres in diameter), and their genome consists of RNA instead of DNA (as also happens with HIV). Furthermore, the genome is especially large by comparison with other viruses, up to three times as big as that of the HIV virus and twice the size of that of the flu virus. SARS-CoV-2, for instance, has 30,000 units, three times more than HIV and twice as many as influenza. Partly because of this, coronaviruses are not easily transmitted by air because they can't travel great distances owing to their weight. However, they can survive for several hours on all kinds of surfaces (with an average of up to three days in some cases), so it's believed that a good many infections occur when a person has contact with one of these microbe havens and then touches a mucosa (mouth, eyes, etc.), thus giving the virus access to the inside of the organism. This is why one of the main recommendations for avoiding infection by coronavirus is washing one's hands well and very often.

Although this was initially controversial, there is now evidence that some coronaviruses, such as the SARS-CoV-2, can also be transmitted through the air, since it has been shown that they can travel up to five metres in tiny droplets, expelled by an infected person when they breathe or cough, and still remain infectious. This could explain why contagions are higher in poorly ventilated rooms, where the floating viruses can accumulate over time, and why face masks can be useful to reduce the risk. It is not clear at the moment which percentage of infections by coronaviruses happen through contact and which through air diffusion.

One interesting characteristic of coronaviruses is that they are among the few RNA viruses with a system for keeping genetic information intact. This is both good and bad news. Since many viruses don't have these error-correcting mechanisms, they can quickly take on mutations, which gives them an evolutionary advantage (because, perhaps after mutation, some viruses can infect more effectively, or survive longer, and so on). Coronaviruses have a more stable genome that amasses few changes. This means that they mutate less (by comparison, for example, with the flu virus or AIDS), which makes it possible to design better vaccines or treatments. On the other hand, though, it means that antivirals that destroy viruses by introducing extra mutations, and are thus very effective in combating some infections, don't work with coronaviruses.

Coronaviruses mainly come from bats and certain rodents, animals in which the viruses can reproduce without making them sick, in most cases. A few dozen viruses from this family are already known, but only seven that cause disease in humans. Four of them account for 20–30 per cent of all colds, and three more new ones, coming from bats (SARS, MERS, and COVID-19), cause serious respiratory infections.

SARS: the coronaviruses enter the scene

SARS (severe acute respiratory syndrome) was the first virus-caused epidemic of the twenty-first century, and also the first of the three big diseases caused by coronaviruses. It began in 2002 in southern China and infected more than 8,000 people around the world with a final death toll of approximately 800 (a mortality rate of 9–10 per cent). There were cases in twenty-nine countries, although the great majority were concentrated in China, Hong Kong, Taiwan and Singapore. Other than these, only Canada had a major outbreak. The epidemic was considered to be over by the summer of 2003, although isolated cases have been seen since then.

From the outset, its swift form of contagion and considerable aggressiveness led to fears that mortality would be very high. Fortunately, the epidemic didn't last long, and the consequences were much less tragic than envisaged in the early estimates, largely because of the confinement decreed in the most affected cities. Although there are no guarantees that we will never see another major outbreak, or even pandemic, it ceased to be an urgent health alert in 2003.

Panic hotel

SARS is an example of how an outbreak of an infectious disease can spread fast in a matter of days. Just one person who was in the wrong place at the wrong time was responsible for spreading the virus to every corner of the world and thus setting off the pandemic.

It's known that an infected Chinese man spent a night in Hong Kong's Metropole Hotel in 2003. There, he came into contact with other travellers who spread the virus to their countries of origin, among them Vietnam, Canada, the United States and Ireland. And this wasn't the end of the outbreak. When the sick people were admitted to hospital, they kept infecting others (for example, one of the hotel guests infected 116 people in a Hong Kong clinic). One passenger on a plane infected twenty-two others taking the same flight. A German who hadn't even been near the Metropole Hotel was infected in a Singapore hospital, so the disease arrived in his country shortly afterwards.

It's been possible to go back even further when tracing the origin of the pandemic. It seems that SARS started in rural zones and was transported to the city of Guangzhou by a farmer who infected many people in the hospital where he was admitted. One of the doctors at the hospital went to a wedding in Hong Kong, and that's how it all began.

SARS is caused by a coronavirus called SARS-CoV. Although it's known that it comes from bats, the path it took in order to make the leap to humans is yet to be discovered. The symptoms of the infection are similar to those of flu, with very high fever. It can be spread when an infected person coughs or sneezes and, in particular, by having contact with a contaminated surface and rubbing the eyes or touching the mouth. So far, there's no vaccine or cure, although several options have been studied. It's been found that griffithsin, a protein extracted from an alga, is highly effective in protecting laboratory mice from SARS, but studies with humans have never been carried out.

It was Dr Yi Guan, a virologist from the University of Hong Kong, who first pinpointed the locus of SARS-CoV in a Chinese animal market, in the spring of 2003. When the virus reappeared at the end of the same year, Guan suggested killing all the wild civet cats sold in the market, since he'd noticed that they were infected and he therefore thought they might have been the bridge between bats and humans. The government listened to him and it's possible that the strategy succeeded, as the virus has been under control since then, except for small outbreaks like that of 2004 when six scientists working with SARS-CoV were infected in a laboratory. Research in the field of SARS was drastically cut once the disease had ceased to be a global health problem, which is why the efforts to find a vaccine, or a successful treatment never came to fruition.

MERS, or camel sickness

In 2012, a new, serious respiratory syndrome caused by coronavirus appeared and, this time, after the disease had been called Middle East Respiratory Syndrome (or MERS), the microbe responsible for it was given the name of MERS-CoV. Like SARS, it can present a great array of symptoms, ranging from a cold to a fatal illness. The first outbreak was seen in Saudi Arabia, and contagion came from camels, although the bat was once again the origin of the virus.

Except for an outbreak in South Korea, MERS has remained quite localized in the Arabian Peninsula and has only affected some 2,500 people (a few hundred cases every year since the first outbreak), which is why it has received little attention at the global level. Yet mortality is quite high, some 35 per cent, or a total of 886 victims. Once again, there's no vaccine or effective drug against MERS-CoV, and treatment aims at reducing the intensity of the symptoms.

COVID-19 changes everything

Coronaviruses took centre stage again in early 2020 when it was announced that an outbreak of a new respiratory disease had been detected in China. It was soon found that the culprit was another virus of the family and very similar to that causing SARS. The outbreak began in the Wuhan zone, in a way that wasn't unlike what happened with SARS but, this time, it couldn't be contained so it ended up causing a pandemic. The main reason for this is that SARS-CoV-2, the virus causing the disease, which was eventually named COVID-19, spreads quickly, partly because the people infected by it are contagious for a lengthy asymptomatic phase. Unlike its close relatives, SARS-CoV-2 is more infectious, most probably because those who have the virus expel larger amounts of it in droplets of saliva. However, it has an average mortality rate that is lower by comparison with the other two more aggressive coronaviruses. Studies carried out so far suggest that the figure is about 1 per cent.

Like other coronaviruses, SARS-CoV-2 has a special predilection for lung cells (and therefore presents respiratory symptomology) but those aren't its only targets inside the body. Like the SARS virus, SARS-CoV-2 adheres to a protein called ACE-2 to get inside human cells. ACE-2 exists not only in the lungs but, in smaller quantities, in many other organs as well, including the intestines, walls of blood vessels and the brain. In some cases, the virus might affect these other tissues, doing less damage and remaining there, perhaps 'dormant', waiting for a chance to reappear later on. There's no conclusive proof yet that this is what happens but, for the time being, the theory can't be discarded.

Owing to this ability to attack different tissues, COVID-19 can present very different symptoms, ranging from loss of the senses of taste and smell (one of its most frequent manifestations, affecting up to 30 per cent of infected people), confusion (perhaps due to its effects on nerves and brain cells) to thrombosis (blood clots), as it also damages the walls of blood vessels. Most cases of COVID-19 are mild or don't even show symptoms, but around 15 per cent are severe and may require hospitalization and oxygen. Only 5 per cent progress to a critical life-threatening stage that needs to be treated with artificial ventilation. Less known at this point are the long-term side effects that might be experienced by those who survive the disease. These could be temporary or maybe even lifelong. Complications, especially in severe and critical cases, may include lung fibrosis, a serious condition that can compromise respiratory capacity. Lasting fatigue isn't unusual either, but this seems to disappear eventually. There are also indications that some survivors may develop diabetes, as the virus destroys insulin-producing cells in the pancreas. In sum, the full extent of the consequences of COVID-19 will only be known after years of observation and study.

It's still not known exactly why COVID-19 is fatal in some patients, while others can be infected without showing any symptoms at all. It's highly possible that genetic determinants exist that are specific to each individual, and this is one area that's now being studied. The immune response has some bearing on the matter. Indeed, a more aggressive reaction, typical of young, healthy people, can set off what's known as a 'cytokine storm', an extreme response that can end up damaging tissues and causing death. In this regard, it's been observed that drugs (such as corticoids) that inhibit this response and reduce the associated inflammation can increase the survival chances of the most critically ill patients. For example, dexamethasone, a cheap, well-known corticoid, has shown a reduction in mortality of up to 30 per cent (a similar response has also been observed with other anti-inflammatory drugs). Some studies observe that thrombosis can also be a decisive factor in COVID-19 mortality rates and, accordingly, recommend the use of drugs (anticoagulants, for example) as a preventive measure with some seriously ill patients. But the fact of the matter is that it's not yet known for sure how SARS-CoV-2 kills, despite the many autopsies that have been carried out. The deaths are clearly not only due to lung damage. It may be that a combination of effects is involved, and the decisive factor will vary from one patient to another.

Although it was originally thought that children didn't become infected, and that the most serious cases were only seen in elderly people or those with pre-existing pathologies, it's now known that the risk of infection is more or less the same for all ages (but there might be differences according to gender, as it seems that men are more susceptible), and that young patients can die too, although this is very rare. However, it's also apparently true that children and young adults normally develop a less severe condition (or show no symptoms) and this is what makes it appear that they are less susceptible to catching the disease. In any case, it's believed that they are probably just as contagious as adults are because the amount of virus in their system is similar, regardless of the lack of symptoms, which could increase the chances of their inadvertently spreading the virus.

Interestingly, epidemiological and mathematical studies have concluded that COVID-19 is usually transmitted by 'super-spreaders', people who release a higher viral load than others and can therefore infect a large number of people simultaneously. This would mean that most people with COVID-19 wouldn't pose a great danger to others, and only a select few would act as 'nodes of amplification' of the disease. The problem, of course, is finding a way to identify who the super-spreaders might be so they can be rapidly isolated. There is no clear indication yet of whether children may or may not act as super-spreaders, which makes it difficult to decide which specific precautions need to be taken in schools. Although initial data suggested that viral transmission in these environments was low, most countries adopted severe measures (reduced class numbers, social distancing, reduced teaching times, hybrid systems that include remote teaching, open-air classrooms, stable 'bubbles' of students that would only interact among themselves, etc.) when schools reopened for the 2020/21 academic year.

Nor is there any certainty about how the virus reached humans. A virus akin to SARS-CoV-2 is believed to have been circulating among bats for decades. There has therefore been no genetic manipulation or anything raising suspicions that this is a virus created in a laboratory, as some people initially suggested (a notion that was immediately discarded once it was possible to read the virus's genome, which showed that there was nothing strange about it). What is not clear is how it made the leap from bats to humans. The original theory was that this had occurred in a Wuhan wildlife market, probably because of another animal that had acted as an intermediary (the pangolin was suggested, although there were other options as well). An alternative hypothesis is that it could have escaped from an important virology laboratory in the area due to a lack of proper controls. Although this is possible, it isn't very likely (the security measures in these laboratories are very stringent, as I explain elsewhere), and there's no credible information that supports this scenario. Animals don't seem to play an important role in the spread of the disease, apart from the initial outbreak. It's been shown that monkeys, hamsters, ferrets and cats (but not dogs) can also catch SARS-CoV-2, but, so far, there's no evidence that any of these animals have infected a human.

In any case, it's highly possible that the virus was circulating earlier than people think. The first cases might have appeared in October or November 2019, and it would seem that there were infected people outside China in the early months of 2020, before the outbreak was announced. Or even before that. The fact that most people would have had no symptoms or might have shown a response that could have been mistaken for the flu (then at the peak of its yearly season) explains why the new disease could have progressed unnoticed until it reached a certain number of cases. It's difficult to trace the disease back to the first cases, but clues are coming from the study of wastewater samples. Parts of the genome of the virus (particles that aren't 'active' viruses, so they can't infect other people) can be expelled in faeces and are later detected in samples from sewers, using a test similar to the one that detects the virus in the blood (known as PCR) and thus allows diagnosis of the infection. Retrospective analyses of these samples are currently being carried out and are helping to map the spread of the virus. Knowing exactly who the first people affected by the virus were, and what path it took, might help us to understand where and how it originated, but there's no guarantee that we will ever unearth all the information.

How to stop the virus

As happens with the other coronaviruses, there's no vaccine and no treatment available to combat SARS-CoV-2, and the only option is to deal with the symptoms as they appear, in order to give the body's defences enough time to end up defeating the virus by themselves. As I said, this may involve resorting to mechanical ventilation if the patient's lungs are badly infected and not enough oxygen is reaching the bloodstream, as well as giving anticlotting drugs and administering corticoids to reduce inflammation and an excessive immune response.

The gravity of the crisis has led to coordinated efforts at the international level, and tests are now being carried out with several drugs that might attack the virus. In March 2020, the WHO began a clinical trial called Solidarity in which about 100 countries joined together to study the four treatments that are believed to have the most chances of succeeding in limiting the progression of the virus once the infection starts: remdesivir, lopinavir+ritonavir, lopinavir+ritonavir plus interferon beta and hydroxychloroquine. In the UK, the RECOVERY trial tested lopinavir+ritonavir to reduce the viral load, but it also includes dexamethasone, azithromycin (a commonly used antibiotic), the anti-inflammatory tocilizumab and hyperimmune plasma (obtained from the blood of patients who have high levels of antibodies against the virus). This trial was the first to show that dexamethasone reduced mortality in the most severe cases, as mentioned before.

One of the first drugs to be proposed as potentially effective in stopping SARS-CoV-2 replication was hydroxychloroquine (or its variant chloroquine), which is normally associated with the treatment of malaria. Some preliminary tests suggested that it could limit reproduction of the virus, but a study published in *The Lancet* in May 2020 found not only that it had no positive effect either on the duration or the seriousness of the disease, but that it could actually increase mortality. Only a few weeks later, it was found that this article was seriously flawed (it seems that a company involved in processing the information had falsified most of the data) and it was withdrawn. However, in early June, a more rigorous study finally demonstrated that chloroquine derivatives were of no use whatsoever in curing or ameliorating COVID-19. So, at present, no data exist to support the use of these drugs as treatment. Yet, despite the absence of reliable positive information, chloroquine was being administered routinely in many hospitals around the world, and even the US president, Donald Trump, announced that he was taking it as a prophylactic because some people believed it could be particularly useful in stopping the virus at the early stages of infection. However, this was also disproved in a study published in June. Moreover, the fact that hydroxychloroquine can have significant side effects, from arrhythmia to liver problems, should be taken into consideration. In short, there is no justification for using it with COVID-19 patients.

At the end of April 2020, the pharmaceutical company Gilead announced that its drug remdesivir reduced the duration of the disease and, later, it was shown to have some effect if given in the early days after infection. Remdesivir is an antiviral that was developed to treat Ebola (but had been found not to work) and it had been shown to affect RNA viruses like those causing SARS and MERS. Its use was immediately authorized in the United States and Japan for the more seriously ill patients, although not all the data had been published at the time, and neither had there been any independent studies to verify the results. But the findings were eventually published and, in June, remdesivir was approved for use in Europe as the first drug shown to have a direct impact on SARS-CoV-2, in particular by reducing the duration of the disease (from fifteen to eleven days, on average), which is a highly beneficial effect in the most severe cases. Nevertheless, it should be noted that remdesivir has some serious side effects, especially with regard to liver function. Moreover, it has to be administered intravenously, and it's expensive, which means that it can't be given routinely to all COVID-19 patients. Controversially, WHO's Solidarity Trial showed in October 2020 that remdesivir actually had no effect in improving survival or length of stay in hospital. Preliminary data suggest that lopinavir+ritonavir may also fall into this category, but more information is needed. Other than these drugs, very few other options are being studied. Hence, the main hope for stopping the pandemic is the vaccine.

The vaccine race

More than 300 possible vaccines were being studied simultaneously in 2020, the highest figure ever recorded for any disease. Many were at different stages of clinical trials in a few months. Indeed, by May 2020, twelve were in the early phases and, in June, three had already progressed to Phase III clinical trials (this number increased to nine in September, with six more in Phase II). Among them is a vaccine produced by Oxford University (ChAdOx1 nCoV-19), which uses another virus to transport parts of SARS-CoV-2 to cells of the immune system. The pharmaceutical company involved in the study was so certain that this vaccine would be successful that it had already started producing doses of the vaccine in mid-June, with a view to having them ready for distribution as soon as all the trials are completed.

The first vaccine to come up with positive results was that being developed by the company Moderna in the United States. An initial trial with only eight patients showed that the vaccine generated antibodies that slowed the virus when studied in the laboratory. Another fairly well-advanced vaccine (Ad5-nCoV) was based on a similar idea and was studied in China with early tests that look encouraging. The government was so confident that this vaccine was going to be successful that it skipped Phase III trials and it was approved for limited use (for the military only). This prompted concerns about safety and the ethics of the decision, since the partially tested vaccine is to be given to a large population without clear guidelines about consent. A few weeks later, Russia announced that it was also registering its vaccine before completing phase III trials, sparking a competition between countries that was compared to the race to the moon. Most scientists have warned that vaccines should only reach the general public when all safety and efficacy tests are completed. An alternative point of view proposed a 'compassionate use' of experimental vaccines to try to reduce the alarming mortality rates. This was opposed by many, who argued that if any not fully tested vaccine were to fail or cause serious side effects, it could be an important blow for vaccination efforts worldwide.

These vaccines I have just described are the most promising at the moment. However, it very much remains to be seen whether any of them will end up being useful, because several phases of the studies still need to be completed with increasing numbers of patients. It's important that simultaneous efforts should be made with as many candidate vaccines as possible because, usually, most of them (up to 80 per cent) don't get through the final clinical trials. In other words, the vaccines that seem most promising in laboratory studies, or in the early stages with volunteers, aren't necessarily the ones that will end up triumphing. It should also be stressed that, rather than using proteins to generate the response, which is the usual procedure, the vaccines that have passed the first trials have employed genetic material from the virus (which, once inside the body, is taken up by human cells in order to produce the viral protein and, thereby, to activate antibodies). So far, no vaccine of this type has been administered on a large scale and, as a result, there's some uncertainty about how these new ones might work.

If things move very fast, the vaccines might appear around twelve to eighteen months after the beginning of the first laboratory experiments (to which must be added the time required to produce enough doses, a quantity that, in this case, could be large). Normally, though, this process takes years, a minimum of four or five and, in many cases, it could drag on for decades. In view of the efforts that have been made and the preliminary results, it was calculated that a candidate vaccine to combat COVID-19 might be approved for general use by the end of 2020 or early in 2021, if the process is speeded up to the maximum. And, of course, if no unforeseen problems emerge. If the vaccine that's first to the post is one of the types based on genes, the production phase (the longest) might be much quicker than it would be if it were necessary to use proteins, but it would also require more effort in setting up the factories to produce it, since the technology is newer. The phases of production, distribution and administration are likely to take many months to reach the goal of immunizing enough people to achieve minimal herd immunity (at least 50–80 per cent of the world's population). It seems that, only then, will we be able to control COVID-19 and downgrade its status as a pandemic disease. Some observers forecast that this will take most of 2021, with a full return to normalcy perhaps in 2022.

In the attempt to achieve this goal, and perhaps even accelerate the final outcome, millions of dollars are being invested to produce the vaccine (the WHO alone initially collected $8 million for this and to test drugs, and many countries and foundations are doing their bit). All efforts are being made to ensure that the process is completed as quickly as possible, and this could mean skipping some of the safety or effectiveness tests, a sacrifice that's believed worth making in order to gain a few months. The result might be a first vaccine that doesn't give complete protection but, even if it only worked for 60–70 per cent of the people to whom it's administered, it would be deemed useful. Other vaccines coming later might be more effective, and the combination of them all could perhaps be what will make it possible to protect most of the population in the long run.

The future of the pandemic

At the time of writing, the COVID-19 pandemic hasn't ended and the course it might take isn't clear. An initial outbreak becomes an epidemic and then a pandemic if the chances of contagion are very high. This is more likely to happen when we are talking about an unknown microbe because no one is immune to it yet. As I have said, when a microbe enters the body for the first time, a response is generated to neutralize it. This includes the production of antibodies, and the cells that produce them remain 'trained' and can respond more efficiently if this or another similar virus infects us again, thus preventing us from getting sick. The same response can be achieved with a vaccine, which spares us from suffering the symptoms of the infection and succumbing to the threats they pose. But, as we've seen, the process of obtaining a vaccine is lengthy, taking months and sometimes even years, and it's not likely to be ready in time to stop the first outbreak of a new disease.

But throughout the history of humanity, there have been dozens of pandemics that have, ultimately, been brought under control. This is nothing new. Measles, polio, rubella and smallpox, to give some well-known examples, are diseases that also caused pandemics in their day but have now ceased to be a problem thanks to the fact that we've developed herd immunity against the viruses responsible for them, mainly because of mass vaccination campaigns. Will the same thing happen with COVID-19? It's too early to tell, but everything suggests that the outcome could be similar in this case too.

What seems most likely is that the coronavirus that causes COVID-19 won't ever go away by itself. It will almost certainly be with us from now on, just as we still coexist with the measles and flu viruses, and the other coronaviruses. As long as we don't have a vaccine, it will keep infecting people, but ever more slowly because the population will be more resistant (but this process is very gradual given that only 5–10 per cent of the world's population had developed antibodies by the summer of 2020). This can eliminate one of the main problems, namely overburdened hospitals, as happens when there are too many cases all at once. In these circumstances, seriously ill patients can't get the full treatment they need, and the mortality rate rises. In the early stages of a pandemic, it's essential, then, to make sure that the cases are spread out over time and that large numbers of people don't turn up *en masse* in emergency departments. As we've seen, the most effective measure is confinement, which has worked very well in flattening the curve of contagion in countries where it's been strictly applied, such as those in Southern Europe. In the UK, for instance, the lockdown rules were not as stringent, and the reduction in the number of cases was much slower.

But even when contagion levels drop after the first phase of the pandemic, it's necessary to remain alert because the virus will still be circulating for a long time. For instance, although most of Europe had achieved low levels of daily contagions by June 2020, the pandemic was still rampant in Russia, India, the United States, Brazil and most of the Americas. With a virus as contagious as SARS-CoV-2, this means that a second wave (and a third, a fourth, and so on) can happen any time, as we've seen with earlier pandemics.

Thus, in this phase of the pandemic, the danger appears in the form of new, practically inevitable outbreaks brought on by increased mobility. They already started to appear in early summer in the countries that were first affected, especially in Asia and Europe, and in some of these places they quickly turned into a second wave. The most prudent course in these circumstances would be to keep restricting certain risky situations such as long-distance travel or crowd-pulling events, at least for a time. However, this conflicts with the need to reactivate everyday life in order to minimize the economic impact of the pandemic, especially at the start of the summer holiday season in the northern hemisphere, and health risks may need to be taken if the economy is to be prioritized.

One of the more plausible scenarios is that a slower rate of contagion will possibly continue in successive waves while we wait for the vaccine and, as a result, the numbers of immune people will slowly keep rising. But, unfortunately, there would be a price to pay when we are talking about a disease that's fatal for a fraction of those who are affected. According to some estimates, between 50 and 70 per cent of the world's population would eventually have been infected if proper measures hadn't been taken in advance. If we assume that the mortality rate of the virus is around 1 per cent, this would have led to some 40 million deaths if lockdown measures hadn't been applied worldwide, which would have placed COVID-19 close to the list of great plagues suffered by humanity. This could still happen if the vaccine is delayed and risky situations aren't avoided. The key, in these situations, will always be to make sure that contagion doesn't affect such large numbers of people before a vaccine is ready.

At the time of writing, there have been more than 30 million confirmed cases of COVID-19, with almost a million deaths officially caused by the disease. However, the actual

First-class passports

One strategy that's been proposed for keeping the COVID-19 pandemic in check is to create an 'immunity passport', which would make it possible to identify people with antibodies against the virus. The theory goes that, supposedly unable to become reinfected or to infect other people, they could lead a normal life. Identifying them would be achieved with serological tests that would specifically measure these antibodies. There already are fast serological tests, but they are quite imprecise and there aren't enough to cover the whole population, which would be necessary in this case. At the same time, it's not actually clear whether everyone who has antibodies would be wholly protected against the virus or how long this immunity will last. Moreover, the idea raises a series of ethical problems: we would be defining a group of premium citizens who'd have more freedoms than the rest. This could give rise to inequalities and even lead to risk-behaviour (people who want to get infected in order to get the passport, for example). All these factors, plus the logistical problems, have been sufficient to prevent it from being implemented anywhere and, indeed, the WHO advised against it.

numbers are likely to be much higher, since many countries weren't carrying out enough tests or recording the casualties rigorously enough. Serological studies (measuring the presence of antibodies in blood) around the world in the first half of 2020 estimated that the percentage of population that had been in contact with the virus was at least ten times higher than the numbers reported. This means that 90–100 million people could have had COVID-19 by June 2020. Similarly, excess mortality (the number of deaths above the five-year average for those months) indicates that the numbers of victims of the disease would by then have been closer to a million (which would fit with the ~1 per cent mortality rate estimated for the virus). Given the fact that the peak of the pandemic had probably not been reached by the autumn of 2020, these numbers could more than double before everything is over.

What lies ahead for SARS-CoV-2

Luckily, SARS-CoV-2 isn't able to vary fast. In the first six months, only twenty mutations were detected and none of them had significantly affected the virus's behaviour. This means that the immunity it generates could last for months or years and – who knows? – maybe even forever, because the specific antibodies will continue to recognize it. Based on what happens with other coronaviruses, the most plausible scenario is protection that will be good for one or two years, but this still needs to be confirmed. The first scientific papers published on the matter indicated that the organism produces a considerable number of high-quality antibodies: first, the fast response type, IgM (immunoglobulin M) and then, a little later, more lasting antibodies called IgG (immunoglobulin G). This process can be measured with serological tests, which are quicker but also less reliable than the RT-PCR tests that directly detect the presence of the virus and are mainly used for diagnosis (see box on p. 146).

However, reports have indicated that reinfection may be possible in certain cases, which would mean that having the disease gives only incomplete immunity to some patients. The few cases confirmed so far suggest that, although reinfections are so far quite rare, it is not clear what percentage of previously infected individuals could actually be susceptible to them. There have also been conflicting studies with regard to the number of infected people who produce protective antibodies. Some say that up to 95 per cent of the cases, including the mildest, show a good immune response, while others venture that the figure would be much lower, especially for those who showed no symptoms. And the extent to which these antibodies are effective isn't clear either. Finally, it is also unknown what role the cells of the immune system that don't need antibodies to perform their function play in the protection, although they seem to be significantly activated in response to SARS-CoV-2. The matter of immunity triggered by the virus is, then, one of the issues that has raised most questions, and it will only be resolved after months of study.

The upshot of all this is that we don't know for sure at the moment how the pandemic will evolve, especially when we factor in the uncertainty about when a large enough proportion of the population will have access to a vaccine. SARS-CoV-2 could become a cyclical virus, like flu, which returns every season. One argument that supports this hypothesis is the fact that high temperatures and humidity decrease (but don't suppress) the rate of infection, probably because the virus doesn't survive as long when airborne or on surfaces. This could lead to cycles of safer summers but an increased risk of outbreaks in autumn and winter until the vaccine grants us the needed immunity.

Once a good part of the population has acquired immunity, it could turn into a virus that causes little more damage than the common cold. The antibodies generated in the first infection (or by the vaccine) might not stop the virus completely, but they could make it more or less innocuous. In fact, some theories postulate that another coronavirus called OC43, which, at present, only causes colds, might also have set off a serious pandemic like that of COVID-19 when it first appeared. This wasn't noticed at the time because it was confused with the flu pandemic of 1889–90 which killed many people. The rest became immune and partly resistant, so the virus was reined in and it caused no more serious pandemics thereafter. Finally, SARS-CoV-2 might behave like the virus that causes SARS and keep appearing from time to time in small serious outbreaks in areas where immunity is lower, but without affecting the rest of the world. We will have to wait a few more months before we can see which path SARS-CoV-2 is most likely to take.

Lessons from COVID-19: how to manage a crisis

It is not easy to deal with a pandemic in a globalized, hyperconnected society where you can land on the other side of the globe in a matter of hours, and where information – including false information – is transmitted at the speed of a click. As we will see in Part II, in 2009 we experienced a simulation of such a situation with the A(H1N1) influenza, a new virus that also spread like wildfire, although, in the end, the pandemic was easily brought under control without having to apply strict measures. In that case, we quickly had a vaccine ready (because a basic vaccine against flu was already available), but there was no need for mass immunizations. However, we knew that this wouldn't always be the case and, indeed, the next pandemic was brought by a virus when not enough research into a vaccine had been done. We've failed to make the most of recent opportunities to design a global action plan against pandemics, one that could, perhaps, have been led by a single entity guided by leading experts and including factors ranging from the most basic research (on potential vaccines and antivirals for the likely suspects) through to guidelines for public health responses. This would certainly have been the ideal situation. Lacking that, we've had to leave the decision-making to individual governments, with all the dangers involved in having to improvise and not having enough resources ready to face the demands in a situation of acute crisis like the one we saw at the start of this pandemic.

When a new virus appears, a quick well-coordinated response is needed until we are fully cognizant of the scope of the disease it causes. Unfortunately, many countries botched the first response to COVID-19, unnecessarily delaying measures that were later found to be essential in slowing the outbreak. Furthermore, public management of the crisis has created bewilderment, distrust and paranoia. There are always some who believe that everything is the plot of some country that's wanted to produce a virus in a laboratory. We need to ensure that this kind of thinking remains marginal, and that the population listens to people who really know about the situation. It's therefore necessary to have a well-thought-out communication strategy and, if possible, one that uses just a few reliable sources of information backed up by the authorities and the media.

What information should be given, and how, must also be discussed. Transparency is essential (SARS was made worse because of the Chinese government's initial attempts to conceal it, and it seems that the same thing may have happened with COVID-19, up to a certain point), but also important is the question of how to make the information available. Some data, dished out to the public in a sensational form by media outlets avid for news to attract readers, don't contribute anything; indeed, on the contrary, they can be harmful. One example is the folly of hoarding masks, toilet paper and other materials thought to be essential, which leads to many places running out of these items, so those who really need them can't obtain them. Another problem is the sense of improvisation conveyed by political leaders who have shown that they lack a clear and agreed-upon strategy for coping with this kind of problem. This spawns mistrust and fear.

For instance, the UK prime minister, Boris Johnson, announced at the beginning of the pandemic that the policy was to allow people to become infected. The reasoning was that, since the mortality rate was very low, most people would recover from the illness and remain immune, which would immediately slow the spread of the virus. Although this strategy of opting for herd immunity has a certain logic, it didn't last very long because the exponential increase in serious cases threatened rapidly to overwhelm the hospitals, which would have greatly increased the mortality figures. In the United Sates, President Donald Trump wasted precious time in the early weeks, claiming that everything was under control and adopting only mild measures, as he was giving priority to protecting the economy. As a result, the United States was among the countries recording the highest numbers of deaths in the first wave. Many other leaders also responded clumsily and, accordingly, the pandemic was soon out of control, for example in Southern Europe, one of the areas most affected in the first wave. By contrast, some Asian countries, perhaps better prepared, thanks to their experience with previous serious epidemics like SARS, were able to flatten the curve of infection quite effectively by applying rapid detection procedures and isolating infected people and their contacts.

However, the experts were also uncertain as to which measures were most effective, and this only added to the confusion. For example, in the United States the CDC recommended against closing schools, while in most other countries it had already been decided that this was one of the first measures that needed to be taken. Something similar happened with masks, which weren't recommended at first (since they give little protection against a virus that doesn't travel far by air) but, later, were thought to be useful if a large proportion of the population wore them (especially to avoid contagion from coughing or spitting by people who were infected but still showed no symptoms). All this shilly-shallying created confusion and mistrust in the public. The WHO has also been harshly criticized for not acting swiftly enough at the beginning and not leading the way. However, the actual executive power of the WHO is minimal, and its advisory role is often ignored. The political pressures to which the organization is subjected (including the threat of withdrawing the funds necessary for its survival, as the United States eventually did) also limits its independence and the impact of its actions.

The figures will need careful analysis when we have the benefit of a little more distance to know which actions were most appropriate and which didn't work, so we can respond better in future. But even with the partial data we have before the end of the pandemic, it would seem clear that the earliest possible isolation of the main loci of infection, and even closing countries, is the method that works best. Fast, forceful action, imposing quarantines and confinement and monitoring borders comprise the most effective response until we have vaccines or drugs. This is why it's so important to be able to count on the cooperation and support of the whole population, since everyone has a part to play if we are going to be able to stop, or at least slow, the initial outbreak.

As I hinted before, COVID-19 has also highlighted the difficulty in enforcing rules that make sense from the scientific standpoint but can lead to major social and economic upheavals. This pandemic has demonstrated that strict confinement is an effective measure, but also that it can only be carried out for a short time. Shutting down the economy on the global scale has social consequences that are too serious to prolong for any longer than is necessary. The problem for politicians is to decide just how long this necessary time will be. While scientific advisers want to have the longest confinement possible, economic powers are calling for a resumption of activity, and the sooner the better. Finding a balance isn't easy.

Consequently, a first, what could be called 'control' phase, during which the main aim is to reduce the number of infections at any price in order to prevent saturation of the health system and a large number of victims, leads into a second 'maintenance' phase, now with different priorities. In this second phase, the aim is a progressive return to normal activity, applying minimal security norms (social distancing, shifts, regular disinfection, staggered return to work, and so on), even though the virus is still present in most countries, and the danger of restarting the pandemic remains high.

The aim, then, is not so much trying to avoid a maximum number of new infections, as in the beginning, but to detect and nip in the bud the more-than-possible new outbreaks when they appear so that the successive peaks of contagion are never as high as they were the first time. From the standpoint of social control of the pandemic, it's unlikely that contagion by a disease that's as infectious as COVID-19 will be reduced to zero because the economic costs would be too great and they, too, would have a direct toll in terms of lives lost.

And the next pandemic?

There will be more pandemics in the future. This is inevitable because viruses are constantly evolving and can always appear in a more aggressive version that would end up leaping from animals to humans. If we look at the history of the flu pandemics humanity has suffered, it seems that there's a big one every so often (between thirty and seventy years). The last influenza pandemic of the twentieth century was in 1968 and the first in the twenty-first century was in 2009. The problem is, as Dr Ana Fernández-Sesma, a Spanish virologist who works in the Department of Microbiology at the Mount Sinai Hospital in New York, points out, 'It's impossible to predict a pandemic',[7] or when or where it will appear, or what microbe will cause it. Fernández-Sesma's laboratory is part of one of the distinguished groups studying influenza in the United States, coordinated by the CDC. When, for example, an influenza epidemic appears, the CDC quickly obtains samples and immediately distributes them to laboratories like that where Fernández-Sesma works. There, they are rigorously examined in order to be able to design the best vaccines and treatments as quickly as possible.

'We need to bear in mind that, nowadays, there are better systems of prevention and detection than before, and also excellent coordination among centres', says Fernández-Sesma. 'So, it's possible to try and contain the infection

---

7   This and the following quotes are from an interview by the author with Ana Fernández-Sesma [translation: JW].

earlier.' For example, in 1968, there were no molecular or genome techniques for identifying and keeping track of viruses, and nor did the Internet exist as a means for immediately sending information to scientists around the world. 'Now, we also have antiviral treatments, and a high percentage of the population is vaccinated against influenza, which could provide partial protection against any new strains that might cause a pandemic.' Dr Adolfo Garcia-Sastre agrees with this opinion: 'In 1918, there were no vaccines or antivirals. The vaccine is very useful with adults and children, and antivirals are good both at the preventive level and if used as treatment, especially if they are given when the symptoms first appear.'[8]

The worst pandemics have been caused by viruses that are especially able to propagate and are also very aggressive, as happens with certain versions of the influenza virus. Luckily, this combination isn't at all common but, when it does happen, the virus is very difficult to stop. This century, bird and swine flu have been forestalled on their way to becoming tragedies, precisely because they have only one of these characteristics. The influenza virus, however, happens to be among those with the best chances at present of causing a pandemic. It changes minimally every year, but every so often these genetic mutations happen on a larger scale. That's when we are more susceptible to the revamped virus, and also when there's a risk of a pandemic. Many experts believe that it's only a matter of time before, in one of these big changes, the influenza virus will turn into a 'supervirus' with all the 'powers' necessary to bring about a true health catastrophe. But, as happened with the appearance of serious diseases caused by the coronaviruses, the one that's

8   See footnote 5 on p. 97.

responsible for the next pandemic could be a microbe that catches us off-guard, or maybe a supervirus that doesn't even exist yet.

In any case, we are better protected against pandemics than we were last century, and a disaster of global proportions would be less likely now. But the downside of all these gains is that progress contributes to the propagation of the virus. The ease of travelling from one side of the planet to the other in a matter of hours means that a localized epidemic can evolve to affect the whole world before it's possible to contain it. After the attack on the Twin Towers on 11 September 2001, when all flights in the United States were cancelled for some days, it was observed that the influenza of that season took longer to spread. It's believed that this is due to the important role of planes in propagating the virus. Hence, some people suggest that, if it were possible to stop all air traffic quickly enough, infections would be much more effectively controlled. During the COVID-19 pandemic, most flights were cancelled, and it's believed that this helped to slow down the spread of the disease (and, as a bonus, shorten the flu season).

We need to bear other factors in mind when speaking of the impact of a pandemic, because its social effects go well beyond the immediate health problems, as we've clearly seen with COVID-19. These factors mustn't be overlooked when designing any response. As early as a decade ago, a US government study envisaged that a serious flu epidemic could kill 2 million people in a few months, with another 8 million hospitalized. And, the study pointed out, that wouldn't be the worst of it. The risk of riots and attacks on pharmacies and hospitals to get medicines, or on shops if food is scarce, and on petrol stations too, is very high. If transport truck drivers fell ill or refused to work, the whole country would soon be brought to a standstill. This means that not only protection and medical treatment of the population has to be guaranteed, but also the minimum necessary services must be maintained. Different kinds of privation would lead to several serious problems that would increase mortality. Moreover, if these fears extended to doctors and hospital workers, patients would be worse attended, and a greater proportion wouldn't survive the flu. The impact of the virus would be dramatically magnified, and this part of the problem is difficult to control.

In this regard, a survey carried out in the United States in 2005 revealed that 40 per cent of health workers said they would stay at home if there was a pandemic. A new survey published in 2009 was a little more promising: only 17 per cent confessed that they wouldn't go to work. During the COVID-19 pandemic, however, it turned out that most health workers around the world made a special effort to keep doing their jobs, even though they knew they were running the risk of infection. This might be partly due to

The virus that will come in from the heat

It's believed that variations in influenza viruses that could end up causing the most serious pandemics are more likely to happen in tropical than in temperate zones. In the latter, flu is seasonal and disappears when temperatures rise. In the tropics, however, the viruses are present all year round, which increases the possibility of genetic changes. Moreover, tropical countries tend to be among the poorest, with fewer resources for detection and fast treatment of cases when they appear. To complicate matters even more, humans often live near farm animals. The viruses' leap between pigs, birds and humans greatly increases the risk of the appearance of variations that can make them more aggressive.

the generalized awareness among the whole population, which would also have been important in helping to establish strict confinement regulations in many countries. Social involvement, then, is one of the essential weapons against pandemics, especially those caused by new microbes, since, when this occurs, science tends to take months before it can help.

Where is the 'supervirus'?

Fortunately, the chances of a 'supervirus' – with the characteristics required to cause a really serious epidemic – appearing spontaneously are actually slighter than may seem, at first glance, to be the case. As Dr García-Sastre says: 'Nature selects viruses on the basis of their ability to spread better. The virus that disperses fastest has better chances of survival. So, a virus that kills quickly won't get very far because its transmission isn't very good.'[9]

Logically, what works best for the virus is to keep the infected person alive so that he or she can infect as many people as possible, thus spreading the virus more efficiently. But there are some exceptions to this rule. Subtypes H5 and H7 of bird flu, for example, are more toxic and are found in domesticated birds but not the wild migratory species. This is because they are transmitted better by the former, which live closer together. In this case, the virus isn't stopped if the bird dies quickly because it can move on quite easily because of the proximity of, say, hens in a henhouse. 'The fact that we humans aren't in such direct contact with each other as poultry in a farmyard makes one think that, if a

---

9   See footnote 5 on p. 97.

highly virulent variant appears, it wouldn't be transmitted very effectively', predicts Dr Garcia-Sastre. 'So, the chances of such an aggressive and easily transmittable viral epidemic are normally not high.'[10]

Predicting pandemics with your computer

In November 2008, Google announced that studying the frequency of search queries appearing on its server could determine the onset of flu epidemics. Google Flu Trends was presented as a service that could detect, before the health authorities, the start of the flu season in different parts of the United States.

The principle is simple. When people start noticing symptoms that they relate with flu, one of the first things they do is to look for information online. Google found that, over the previous five years, the increased number of searches containing the word 'flu' neatly coincided with the medical data on the incidence of infection in the United States. WHO experts began studying the practical applications of the tool but, later, it was described as an 'epic failure'.

What would be the ideal conditions for the appearance of a 'supervirus'? Let's imagine that the bird flu virus H5N1 and the swine flu virus H1N1 exchange genetic information. The resulting virus could be as aggressive as the former and as quickly transmitted as the latter. We would then have serious difficulties battling such an organism. H5N1 has been detected in more than sixty countries around the world, while H1N1 has taken a similar path and is also found in

10   See footnote 5 on p. 97.

Asia where H5N1 is more common. The more widespread these two viruses are, the greater the chances that, one day, they will turn up in the same animal. They can also exchange information with viruses that are resistant to the usual drugs, which would endow this theoretical 'supervirus' with a third 'power'. Evidently, the base needn't be an influenza virus. A coronavirus or even one from a family we don't know about, or that we consider to be a 'minor' type could manage to mutate enough to cause serious problems.

Health and economy: an inevitable relationship

It's easy to criticize the pharmaceutical companies for wanting to make money from such a basic need as medicines, but it's also true that they are an essential part of the health system on the global scale.

Here's an example. Before the 2009 influenza pandemic, Novartis was planning to close some of its plants that had been producing vaccines because they weren't profitable. But the sudden high demand from government meant that the vaccines were once again good business. It also allowed companies to invest resources in setting up more units and researching ways of improving the product. Protection can therefore extend to a larger part of the population.

The fact that someone is making a profit means that we can be sure that we'll have the supplies we need if there's a crisis. Hence, economic interest ends up improving healthcare. One example is the race to find a vaccine for COVID-19, in which several pharmaceutical companies are making great efforts and investing large amounts of money. Thanks to their interest in monopolizing the fabulous profits held out by a vaccine of which we will need thousands of millions of doses very quickly, the most likely result is that more than one candidate will get to the finishing line.

How can we prevent the spread?

Is there any way of stopping a pandemic once it's under way? Or can it even be averted before it becomes a pandemic and spreads all over the planet? I have said that possibly the best weapon we have against infection is a vaccine, but it's also true that, when faced with a new virus, it normally takes some months or even years before we can produce one that would be effective. If the next pandemic is a variant of one that's known, for example the influenza virus, then we would almost certainly be quicker in having a defence against it ready for use.

In 2004, before SARS and bird flu activated plans against possible pandemics, the production of a seasonal flu vaccine was some 300 million doses per year. At present the figure has more than doubled. It's believed that, if efforts are coordinated, as many as 2,000 or 3,000 million doses of specific vaccines could be produced in a year, but this would only be enough to provide group immunity to less than half the world's population. And there's little doubt that such a quantity would only be achieved by stopping the production of other vaccines, for example that being developed against seasonal flu, which would have negative consequences and cause an additional number of deaths. Hence, we need to think carefully about how to distribute resources and, in doing so, to bear in mind the fact that the viruses that cause pandemics are different from those that are normally circulating, which means that most of the population has no immunity against the former, as we've seen with SARS-CoV-2. It might happen that two doses of vaccine will have to be given in order to be sure that immune defences are activated, and this would mean halving the number of people who could receive it in any given period.

The group led by Dr Iain Stephenson of the University of Leicester has drawn attention to the fact that at least six months are needed to produce the vaccines necessary to confront a pandemic. Their study calculated that, in this time, the first wave of infections would have petered out by itself but leaving in its wake a large number of deaths if the virus is aggressive enough. Accordingly, the vaccine, for all its great potential in preventing the influenza from continuing to spread, is not very useful as a first line of defence.

Indeed, the 2009 influenza pandemic also demonstrated that, even if a vaccine could be designed quickly, it isn't possible to obtain enough doses for all the people who need them in a reasonably short time. Some estimates suggest that only between 20 and 30 per cent of the world population could be vaccinated in the early months of having a vaccine. We will know more about this when a vaccine against COVID-19 is produced and vaccination begins. This will entail significant differences between rich and poor countries in terms of distribution of the vaccine. The United States, for example, is the country that asked for most doses against the 2009 influenza pandemic. Its orders, and those of a few other rich countries, monopolized the entire world's production for six months. The fear was that if the United States started to distribute the vaccine indiscriminately, many other countries would be left without. Fortunately, in that case the pandemic was stopped before this scenario was played out, but we might have to face it now, with COVID-19, as the United States has announced that it is willing to pay whatever price is necessary to get hold of the first doses, and other countries that have pharmaceutical companies capable of producing the vaccine within their territory are very likely to demand a place at the top of the list (see box). This distribution of doses, defined more by economic criteria than by actual health needs, could have a major impact on the total

Getting in on the ground floor

Which countries should get doses of the vaccine first in a pandemic if, in the beginning, there aren't enough for everyone? Some countries with vaccine producers within their borders will make the most of their advantage. During the 2009 influenza crisis, Holland did a deal with the company Solvay in which it was guaranteed the first 17 million doses produced. But many countries still don't have these production plants on their soil, which places them at a disadvantage if there's a pandemic. In 2009, the United States government invested $1,000 million to increase the production of the traditional vaccines, and an additional $100 million went to a company that produces FluMist, a new kind of anti-influenza vaccine.

At the beginning of this century there were flu vaccine producers in only nine countries. They could cover the demand for vaccines against seasonal flu but not against an influenza pandemic. Hence, new plants were immediately constructed (in Brazil, Taiwan, South Korea, Mexico and elsewhere). Despite these efforts, there aren't enough resources yet for producing many doses of the vaccine in a very short time, or for guaranteeing a just distribution.

In September 2020, the WHO issued a series of guidelines suggesting that COVID-19 vaccines should be distributed fairly among all countries, prioritizing those with more urgent needs. It was the first systematic attempt to set the rules for ethical vaccine distribution in a pandemic, although the WHO doesn't have the power to enforce them.

number of deaths, and in the speed of bringing a pandemic under control.

The other important weapon we have for curbing epidemics is drugs. As I said, the problem is that those we have aren't excessively effective or varied, and the possibilities of having one that would work against a new virus aren't very good. Then again, the experts don't agree over whether antivirals should be given as a preventive measure to those who've been in contact with infected people but haven't yet fallen ill, or whether they should be kept only for those people showing symptoms. Abuse of antivirals could raise the chances of resistances appearing and, in addition, would mean a perhaps unnecessary drain on drug reserves. In the COVID-19 pandemic, we've seen that chloroquine and antiretrovirals (like those used for AIDS) were given to the more seriously affected patients without carrying out the necessary tests beforehand to determine whether they have any effect on SARS-CoV-2. Medical emergency forced a breach of scientific protocol, with serious ethical consequences.

With regard to preparation against a pandemic, the experts advise governments to amass enough doses of the more common antivirals in order to treat the first people who are infected and thus effectively to stop transmission. It's calculated that Western countries have stores of between 220 and 250 million doses of Tamiflu for treating influenza. The United States has a total of 50 million and the WHO only 5 million. If we recall that the 1918 pandemic infected 800 million people, it's evident that these stocks are insufficient and most of those infected in a potential flu pandemic will go untreated. Some people recommend that the stocks should also include a percentage of doses of another antiviral, one that is different from Tamiflu, so that the two types can be given to different parts of the population in order to avoid the appearance of viruses that are resistant to one of the drugs and, if this should happen, an alternative treatment will be available. The obstacle is still the fact that antivirals are expensive to produce, which means that they are out of reach for most developing countries.

It could also be important to use antibiotics for avoiding secondary infections, which, as I've said, can result in a large number of the deaths related to viral infections. In the 1918 influenza pandemic, many deaths were the result of these secondary infections and, accordingly, part of the first line of treatment for COVID-19 includes an antibiotic, azithromycin, just to be on the safe side. And, also with regard to COVID-19, we've seen that simple, widely used drugs (like anti-inflammatories or those that prevent blood clotting) could significantly reduce mortality in the worst cases.

Apart from the vaccine and treatment, other strategic possibilities exist for slowing a pandemic, which depend on the organization and responses of governments, as I've already noted. One of the most effective of these, as we've seen during the COVID-19 pandemic, is swift isolation of those infected (with follow-up of possible contacts) and, at the same time, avoiding gatherings of large numbers of people. When an outbreak of an infectious disease is suspected, it's important to act fast to ban crowded public events, and to close schools, leisure centres and so on. According to the mathematical models used to predict the success of such measures, they are only really useful if taken in the first two weeks after the first cases appear. After that, the virus spreads too widely for the early contagion to be slowed down, and the curve representing the number of people infected rises exponentially, with the risk that an epidemic or a pandemic will be declared.

Another key to controlling a pandemic is early diagnosis: the earlier the cases can be identified, the more effective will be the measures to isolate them and prevent the infection from spreading. Dr Christian Drosten of the Institute of Virology at the University of Bonn designed the first test for diagnosing SARS in 2003. In April 2009, he set about trying to find a more effective diagnosis for the influenza pandemic that was starting in Mexico. This was based on detecting a zone of the virus's DNA that was unique and different from those of other influenza viruses. In less than four days, his team of scientists localized the specific part they needed to identify and then refined the techniques. After that, the basic tests began to be distributed free of charge to hospitals around the world. This is an example of the speed with which new systems of detection can be implemented. We've seen this, too, with COVID-19. In a few weeks, a test for diagnosing the presence of the virus in blood using the technique known as RT-PCR had been designed and, shortly afterwards, there was another test to determine who had antibodies against the microbe. Owing to differences between viruses, a special diagnostic system has to be designed for each pandemic, which is why immediate action is important when a new outbreak is detected.

World health planning must be very conscious of the fact that no risks can be taken. The WHO and governments have the obligation of being ready for the worst-case scenarios, even if they seem improbable. Experts therefore need to discuss what the best response would be from the beginning of a pandemic and make their decisions in keeping with the data that become available at every point along the way, as this will be changing from one week to the next. It's frequently difficult for citizens and even health workers to take in all the factors involved in this process, since they require a high degree of knowledge about the theoretical behaviour of a pandemic.

The consequences of not being ready to confront a possible serious pandemic are too important, so every effort should be made. From this standpoint, stockpiling antivirals is a strategy that many community health experts agree might be correct. Obviously, this means the enrichment of producers of antivirals, but we must also be aware that, without their contribution, we would never be able to confront an aggressive virus if it should appear. The involvement of the pharmaceutical companies in controlling pandemics is both inevitable and essential. Being ready for the worst of cases, even if it never happens, will always be better, from the public health point of view, than not being cautious enough and then being caught unawares by a health crisis for which we aren't properly prepared.

Part II

Major Modern Epidemics

7

Influenza

Flu is a very common disease. Thousands of people suffer from it every year but the great majority recover without problems. It's an infection caused by the influenza virus, with symptoms including high fever, shivers, general aches and pains, headache, coughing and sometimes nausea and vomiting. The virus is often mistakenly blamed for other illnesses. The common cold or gastroenteritis, for example, have very similar though milder symptoms. In these cases, the microbes involved are different. It's probable that many people who think they've had the flu have actually had one of these other infections.

If the flu isn't much more than a heavy cold, why are the experts so concerned about it? The reason is that a certain percentage of those infected can have very grave complications, which can even cause death. Since this is a virus that spreads to a lot of people, the numbers quickly become worrying. In the United States, for example, between 5 and 20 per cent of the population catch the flu every year.

About 200,000 people are hospitalized, and the mortality rate is estimated to be in the region of 36,000. In the United Kingdom, mortality has oscillated between 10,000 and 30,000 per year over the last five years. The annual death rate worldwide is between 250,000 and 500,000, of whom 90 per cent are older than 65, this being one of the two age groups most at risk from serious complications caused by the virus. The other high-risk group is small children. What these two cohorts have in common is a less potent immune system, which makes them especially vulnerable.

Once infected by the influenza virus, people develop antibodies capable of blocking it, possibly for the rest of their lives. This would mean that we would only have the disease once, as happens with measles, if it weren't for one detail: every year, the influenza is caused by a virus that's slightly different from that of the previous season and frequently sufficiently so for it not to be recognized by our defences. This is why we still feel vulnerable to the disease and it's so difficult to find vaccines and treatments that could be used against all the variants that might keep appearing.

Protected forever?

Recent tests with blood from people who survived the 1918 influenza pandemic have shown that, 90 years after being infected by the virus, they still have defences against it. The antibody-producing cells extracted from the blood of these individuals protected mice that were exposed in the laboratory to the 1918 virus.

The experts are always talking about the imminent risk of an influenza pandemic and have continued to warn of this possibility even though people didn't paid much attention to them until, in the spring of 2009, this century's first pandemic broke out and, indeed, it was caused by an influenza virus. Was it really as serious as some people predicted? Is there any way of preventing these pandemics? Or of stopping them once they've started? Could an influenza virus wipe out the human race, as it has been on the verge of doing in other epochs, or is that danger a thing of the past? These and other similar questions were raised in 2009 and, a decade on, reappeared with the century's second pandemic: COVID-19. In what follows, I will try to offer some answers.

The virus's thousand faces

There are three types of influenza virus: A, B and C. The most common is A, which can infect different species, humans among them. In fact, it's the most aggressive of the three. Type B, almost exclusively confined to humans, isn't very common, and C is even less so.

Type A viruses have eleven genes that produce the proteins needed by the virus to divide and infect. These genes are also classified into several 'subtypes' depending on the variations of two of their proteins, *haemagglutinin* (abbreviated to H) and *neuraminidase* (or N). There are sixteen different versions of haemagglutinin (numbered 1 to 16), and nine of neuraminidase (1 to 9). In the 2007–8 season, for example, a virus of the H3N2 subtype was circulating and, in 2009, the seasonal flu was H1N1, like that which caused the pandemic of both that year and the one of 1918. So, even if they have the same Hs and Ns, the viruses can be more or less potent. It's believed that, in general, those with H5 or H7 are the most virulent of all. There are also variants called *strains* within each subtype.

How can the influenza virus keep changing every year,

taking all these forms? One reason is its tremendous ability to traffic in genetic information. Like a kid swapping stickers in the schoolyard, an influenza virus can take a bit of DNA from another virus of the same family and give it some of its own in exchange. The gene collection they both end up with after these 'deals' can be so different from the original ones that the resulting viruses could be regarded as practically new, or at least from the point of view of our immune systems.

ID cards

Here are the classifications of some of the more famous influenza viruses, all of them type A:

Spanish flu (1918): H1N1
Asian flu (1957): H2N2
Hong Kong flu (1968): H3N2
Bird flu (1997–): H5N1
Swine flu (2009): H1N1

The official names of the influenza viruses are normally given as follows: Type / Region where discovered / Strain / Year of discovery (Subtype).

If a virus is called A/USSR/90/77 (H1N1), this means it caused an epidemic in the USSR in 1977, and is of type A, and strain 90, and subtype H1N1.

This 'schoolyard' where viruses meet to do their deals needs clearer definition. One option is us – that is to say, the human body. If two different influenza viruses infect the same person at once, they can exchange genes. But this happens much more frequently in other species. Certain animals act as *reservoirs* or places where viruses accumulate and live for a certain time. In the case of influenza, the reservoirs are birds, in particular, but they can also be pigs. This is possible because most human influenza viruses don't cause serious health problems for the animals they infect, and they can therefore stay with them for a long time without making them sick, thus increasing the possibilities that two or more viruses will end up coinciding.

Animal reservoirs are also the reason why the influenza viruses are never completely eliminated, even when they don't infect humans for months and it seems that they've disappeared off the face of the Earth. Birds and pigs would act as a sort of 'pantry' in which the virus survives as it waits for the right time to make the leap to humans again. The worst influenza pandemics of history were due to viruses coming from birds (as may have happened in 1918), but the possibility that some of them found refuge in pigs before going back to birds and then on to humans hasn't been ruled out either. This could have been the case in 1957 and 1968.

The killer cold

Influenza is transmitted from one individual to another because the virus travels in drops of saliva. Apart from direct contagion – if we are near a sick person who coughs or sneezes – we can also be infected by shaking hands or touching our nose, mouth or eyes after contact with a contaminated surface, since the virus can live outside the body for up to twenty-four hours. After a period of incubation, lasting several days or even a week, the actual illness will begin. We should remember that a person is usually contagious only as long as the symptoms of the disease are present.

We still don't know why the flu can end up being fatal in a small percentage of cases. One theory is that the virus paralyses the body's defences, thus encouraging the appearance of other simultaneous infections like pneumonia brought on by bacteria that, in normal conditions, almost certainly wouldn't have caused any problem. So, in fact, it would be the bacteria that end up killing the sick person. It's been suggested that up to one-third of pneumonia deaths of children under the age of 2 in Africa could be due to influenza. If this theory is confirmed, the statistics for the total number of influenza deaths would rise, as pneumonia is the disease that causes most child deaths: up to 2 million per year.

Death can also result from an opposite effect on our defences, namely the so-called cytokine storm, which can attack the lungs irreversibly. Cytokines are chemical substances released by the body to 'wake up' its defences when an invader appears. If produced in excess, they trigger an inordinate inflammatory reaction with an accumulation of cells and fluids in the wrong places, which can prevent the organs from functioning and, in extreme cases, lead to death. Some influenza viruses (like H5N1, or bird flu, and the 1918 flu) are especially able to set off this reaction, which is why they affect mainly young people with an intact immune system, unlike other kinds of flu viruses that, as I've said, most severely affect people whose defences aren't very active. It's believed that, in some cases, COVID-19 would prompt this reaction, in which case there would be higher chances of serious consequences.

Finally, it's known that a deficient diet can contribute towards worse reactions to the flu virus. Studies using laboratory animals have shown that if their calorie intake is cut by at least 40 per cent, they are more likely to die when infected by the virus. And those that survive take longer to recover. Once again, the reason for this is weakening of the immune system, so it's important that the body is as fit as possible at the start of the flu season.

A winter malady

It's known that flu appears cyclically, so the risk of catching it isn't the same all year round. These outbreaks are seen around the world, following a pattern that's called *seasonal*, punctually beginning in winter and ending around spring-time. Knowledge of this rhythm dates back to ancient Greece and, thanks to this, we can produce vaccines and devise other strategies to lessen the impact.

What makes the flu follow this pattern? According to several studies, the virus is more stable and therefore more infectious when temperatures and humidity are low, or in the conditions of the cooler months. Other contributing factors could be that, in winter, people tend to spend more time in closed spaces than outside, thus facilitating contact and transmission. A theoretical decline in the efficiency of our immune systems due to the cold weather and lack of the melatonin and vitamin D that we get from the sun could also have an influence, but none of these theories explains why there are also cases of flu in tropical climes, so there will cer-tainly be other, as yet unknown, factors.

Yet, the great danger for humans doesn't come from winter flu outbreaks. Sometimes, and totally unpredictably, there's a global pandemic due to a new virus against which we have no immunity. These pandemics don't follow the same pattern, so, for example, the first wave of the 1918 flu in Denmark was at the height of summer. They are usually caused by much more aggressive forms of the virus that are transmitted faster and can have a high death toll. Although the number of casualties left in the wake of the seasonal flu each year is by no means negligible, it can't be compared with the devastation that can be wrought by one of these pandemics when the conditions are in its favour.

Aggressive outbreaks

Only in very specific cases of seasonal flu are there especially aggressive outbreaks that tend to be more akin to the pandemic influenzas. In July 2002, for example, 70 per cent of the 2,160 inhabitants of the town of Sahafata in Madagascar caught the seasonal flu and 27 people died. A series of social and sanitary problems together with an especially cold winter contributed to the high number of cases.

A useful treatment

Humans have been at the mercy of the flu for many centuries. We can't do much more than treat the symptoms and wait for the disease to run its course. Not long ago, we discovered a series of drugs that attack the virus successfully enough to considerably reduce the complications of the infection. These antivirals kill the virus by specifically blocking the proteins that are essential for its survival.

The main treatment against the flu nowadays is oseltamivir – better known by its brand name Tamiflu – which inhibits the activity of the virus's neuraminidase. Star anise, a natural component and one that's not easy to find, is needed to make Tamiflu, so we can't obtain as much as we would like. However, a synthetic form can be used to solve the problem, speed up the production process and make it more efficient.

Zanamivir, marketed under the trade name Relenza, another drug from the same group, is less effective but has fewer side effects. While Tamiflu is a pill, Relenza is administered as a nasal spray. Strange as it may seem, these two very important drugs didn't exist until the very end of the twentieth century. They were publicly presented in 1998 and started to be used in Europe in 1999.

As was to be expected, viruses that survive the drugs have appeared. Until 2007, resistance to Tamiflu was rare but, then, a virus that was circulating at the beginning of the 2008–9 season didn't respond to Tamiflu in 98 per cent of cases when, in the previous season, resistance was just over 1 per cent. Normally these resistant viruses aren't very aggressive, and they are still sensitive to other antivirals so they haven't been a big problem yet, but no one can guarantee they will stay like that in future. The fact that a virus can become resistant to Tamiflu is a serious setback because governments all around the world have been accumulating doses of the drug for years with a view to using them urgently if a pandemic is declared, as I've explained. Research aiming to find new antivirals is now under way, but this is a very slow process, and it's difficult to predict when they will be ready.

One vaccine or many vaccines?

As I said, owing to the virus's ability to change a little every season, there's no vaccine that can provide immunization against all the possible kinds of influenza viruses. It's necessary to design a new one every year. Scientists study which strains are circulating months before the beginning of the season, after which they produce a vaccine against the ones they believe will be seen most often when the cold weather comes, and large-scale production begins as soon as the necessary tests are completed. The whole process can last some six to eight months, from the time when the viruses are identified (usually in early spring) to the moment when the vaccine is ready for use, in about October, just when the first outbreaks are appearing in the northern hemisphere.

Decisions about which vaccine is to be used are made, under supervision, by the Global Influenza Surveillance

Network (GISN), a group with 110 centres distributed around 85 countries; established in 1947, it comes under the auspices of the WHO. The GISN organizes two annual closed-door meetings with scientists and pharmaceutical companies in order to make informed decisions. At one of these (in February) the vaccine for the northern hemisphere is chosen, and, at the other, the one for the south is decided, with a view to their being ready in time to coincide with the arrival of winter in the two halves of the globe.

For all the scientists' efforts, the effectiveness of a vaccine is variable. The success of their choice in 2008, for example, was only 44 per cent by comparison with the 70–90 per cent that was expected of it. This was probably due to an error in prediction when deciding which would be the most prevalent flu strains that year. The result was a higher than usual number of victims of the seasonal flu. Accordingly, some experts call for more transparency and participation at the meetings where the composition of the vaccine is decided, since a wrong choice, as happened in 2008, can have very serious consequences around the world.

The search is still continuing for a possible universal vaccine that could be used year after year without having to change it, but, in order to achieve this, we need to find, first of all, zones in the virus that are conserved without much variation and that, in addition, can induce a powerful immune response. This combination isn't at all frequent, but progress is being made in the field. In April 2009, a group of scientists at the Saint Louis University in the United States announced that they had produced a vaccine designed to thwart a good number of variants of the influenza virus and had tested it with hundreds of volunteers. It was the first clinical test of this kind to be made, but no such 'supervaccine' has yet been made available to the public. Other earlier experiments had managed to block nine kinds of viruses in mice, including that responsible for the 1918 pandemic and that for bird flu H5N1. The results, therefore, seem promising, and one day, perhaps, we'll have a flu vaccine that lasts longer than a year.

The future of humanity depends on an egg

The system for producing the flu vaccine hasn't changed since the mid-twentieth century. First, the virus that the vaccine is meant to be combating is modified in the laboratory so it can reproduce well in a hen's egg. Then, it is injected into as many fertilized eggs as are needed to obtain a large amount of the virus. The antigens are then purified from these cultures and made ready to stimulate the human immune system once they've been injected. Not all the variants of the microbe divide equally well in the eggs, so the speed at which vaccines can be produced varies from one year to the next.

To meet the world's annual vaccine needs, millions and millions of eggs are needed, and these have to be ordered at specialist farms months in advance. This system has an obvious weakness: if, at some point, there's an epidemic of bird flu (or some other disease affecting birds) and a large number of chickens die, the production of eggs required for that season could be insufficient. For some time now, experts have working on safer and more effective ways of obtaining the vaccine. The main aims are to accelerate the production process and to be sure that the maximum number of people will have access to it in case of need.

One option is to use inactivated viruses rather than dead ones, which is the usual procedure. It's considered more dangerous, as the attenuated viruses of the vaccines can themselves cause infections in some cases. The advantage of attenuated viruses is that using them could multiply by 100 the ability to produce vaccines. since the amounts needed to prompt an immune response are much smaller. For each egg, 50–100 doses could be achieved this way, while, in the present system, one or two eggs are needed for every dose.

Other systems that don't depend on hens have also been found, for example vaccines based on cell cultures. In this case, mammalian cells are infected with the virus, which is left in them to reproduce for some days. Then, large quantities of the antigen are purified from the cell fluids. This is a faster, cleaner system that doesn't need a supply of specially prepared eggs, as the virus is cultivated in cells under laboratory conditions. The first vaccine of this kind was approved in Europe at the end of 2007 and, since 2016, cell culture vaccines have been used regularly, although 90 per cent still come from eggs.

Another system is to introduce into plants genes that produce proteins similar to those of viruses. This is achieved by means of cell cultures, using the virus to transport the gene, or producing transgenic plants containing the gene concerned. This way, plants produce the virus protein that is to be used as an antigen. A large amount of protein from its leaves can be purified in a relatively short time. This method is already being tested for vaccines against poliomyelitis, cholera, rabies and flu, among other diseases, but the clinical trials are still in the early phases. At present, only one vaccine generated by this method has been approved, and only for use with chickens.

The danger of bird flu

The first warning of an influenza pandemic in the twenty-first century was the so-called bird flu, caused by one of the most aggressive versions ever seen of the H5N1 virus. It is fatal for 50 per cent of the people it infects and, in the worst cases, can kill in less than two hours. Antivirals are partially effective in slowing the infection, but only if given in the first twenty-four hours. For the moment, the number of casualties caused by the H5N1 virus is low because, fortunately, it's poorly transmitted. It's mainly found in birds and has been passed on to humans on just a few occasions. Contagion has mainly come about because of close proximity to some animal or bird, so the scope of the disease is limited to people who have direct contact with livestock.

It is believed that the origin was ducks in China. The first H5N1 outbreak detected in humans was in 1997, in Hong Kong. Eighteen people were infected and six of them died shortly afterwards. The swift response of the Chinese government, which decided to slaughter nearly 1.5 million chickens and ducks, brought an immediate halt to the infection. H5N1 didn't reappear until 2003 and, at the beginning of 2004, it was found that it had become even more virulent. Months later, its presence was detected in pigs as well, which gave rise to fears of a possible genetic mix with other viruses that would end up producing a more easily transmitted variant. In 2005, H5N1 started to show resistance to amantadine, one of the antivirals that was then being used. Some scientists suspected that this was because Chinese farmers were indiscriminately giving this relatively cheap drug to their chickens so they wouldn't get sick. The danger of a terrible pandemic caused by a vaccine-resistant virus, which could kill millions of people, suddenly seemed to be a not-so-distant possibility.

Between 2005 and 2006, bird flu was front-page news. President George W. Bush announced that the United States would allocate more than $7,000 million to prepare the country for a possible pandemic. The alarm was even greater in early 2006 when it was found that the virus had mutated once again and, as foreseen, could now infect humans more easily. Moreover, birds migrating to warmer climates had spread the virus to countries a very long way from the source of the outbreak, so it appeared in Lagos, Nigeria, and was also, around this time, being detected in Europe, especially in Greece, the United Kingdom, Austria and Germany. It was feared that numerous outbreaks would very soon appear among humans around the world and that little could be done to stop them.

Nevertheless, the H5N1 bird flu peaked in 2006. That year, of the 115 people who were infected, 79 died. In 2007, the figures were 59 dead out of 88 infected and, ever since then, the numbers have fallen, but the reasons for this aren't clearly understood. The virus hasn't totally disappeared, but it has ceased to represent an immediate danger for the time being. In the end, without any human intervention, the feared pandemic didn't happen.

In any case, efforts to prepare for bird flu have continued lest it should again be a problem in future. In 2007, the first vaccine against H5N1 was achieved, produced by Sanofi Pasteur, but it only gave partial protection. Organisms and foundations like the Pasteur Institute, the Wellcome Trust and the Bill & Melinda Gates Foundation launched a programme in 2008 with a view to stimulating research into the weak points of our defences against bird flu, in order to obtain faster results in the areas where they were most needed. The main idea was to coordinate research efforts around the world so as to achieve quicker results, and also to guarantee proper monitoring systems and fast dissemination of information. One of the initiative's recommendations was to stockpile what's called a 'pre-pandemic' vaccine that, made on the basis of what was known about the H5N1 virus, would offer partial protection given that the virus is still changing and it isn't clear whether it will

The name game

Finding the best name for a new disease is complicated. Once, the usual thing was to name it after the country or zone where it was discovered (as happened with Ebola, Marburg and MERS) but now it's considered that this isn't fair to the people living in these places, who might even suffer discrimination. Hence, COVID-19 ended up having this neutral name, which is an abbreviation for 'coronavirus disease of 2019'.

An example of how complicated it is to name new infections is the case of the 2009 flu pandemic. At first, it was called swine flu because of its animal origin. But Israel's deputy health minister asked, as a sign of respect for Jewish and Muslim customs that prohibit the consumption of pork, that the name be changed to 'Mexican flu''. The idea was applauded by farmers around the world. The Dutch were already using the name, but Mexicans, who, unsurprisingly, didn't agree, simply called it 'the epidemic'. Others suggested that it should be called 'North American flu'.

Following a long discussion, the WHO admitted that 'swine flu' wasn't the most appropriate name. After 30 April 2009, it was officially named 'A(H1N1) influenza', a scientific name based on the type of virus responsible, although it wasn't very accurate because it could be applied to many other flu outbreaks. In some places, the epidemic was given the even more incongruous name of 'new flu'.

It wasn't until July 2009 that the WHO found the definitive technical name: (H1N1) pandemic 2009. But despite everything, people and the media kept using a mixture of the earlier names.

ever cause a pandemic. Countries would keep progressively accumulating the vaccine as they've done with Tamiflu. In 2008, the European Commission approved Prepandrix, a vaccine of this type produced by GSK, and the United States and Finland were the first countries to place their orders.

Bird flu no longer has the media interest it aroused at the beginning of the century because it hasn't measured up to the most pessimistic expectations, but we must never forget that the threat still exists. The virus has become endemic in bird populations of countries like Egypt, Indonesia, Bangladesh and Vietnam. This means that it can never be eradicated from these zones, and that it will continue to infect humans from time to time. In mid-2008, the virus was detected in birds of more than sixty countries. Although it seems that it is increasingly less prone to being passed to humans, possible new outbreaks as it keeps moving into other zones cannot be ruled out.

A 2006 study calculated that, if bird flu finally became a pandemic, it could end up infecting between 50 and 80 million people around the world, most of them in developing countries. Given the high mortality rate among those infected, the consequences would be terrible, which is why efforts are still being made to find the best ways of combating it. The fact that fear of bird flu sounded all the alarms in 2005 and obliged us to prepare for a possible pandemic is one of the reasons why the response to the 2009 influenza was so fast and strong.

The 2009 influenza pandemic

The first pandemic this century was influenza, but not of avian origin. It was caused by a virus that's believed to come

The genealogical tree

Genetic analysis of the 2009 pandemic flu virus made it possible to conclude that it is of the A(H1N1) type and a close relative of that which caused the 1918 influenza pandemic. It is believed that pigs became infected then too, but they were resistant and not many died. According to this theory, H1N1 then remained in the world pig population, changing and evolving. After 1998, it would have mixed with an H3N2 human virus as well as a bird flu virus. This triple blend would have infected pigs in Asia, from where it would have spread around the world. Eventually, in 2009, it would have passed to humans again, although it's not known exactly how or where.

from pigs, although it's mixed with bird flu genes and also human strains. The main difference with earlier cases of outbreaks also coming from animals is that, this time, the virus moved very easily among humans and there was no need for direct contact with livestock. And this is why it spread around the globe so quickly.

The story began on 21 April 2009 when the US government announced that, at the end of March, it had detected an 'unusual' outbreak of influenza coming from Mexico. Some sources say it was the Canadian government that was first to alert the Mexican government, because a Canadian citizen who had visited the country presented symptoms of the disease. Whatever the case, when the information was made public, up to 1,000 people were already infected, which made it practically impossible to contain the outbreak. The reason for the delay was that it wasn't easy to identify the newly appeared virus. There was a sudden, strangely high number of patients being admitted to hospitals with respiratory problems, but they were confused with cases of the normal seasonal flu which was already under way (as also happened with the COVID-19 pandemic). One of the few differences was that vomiting and diarrhoea were among the symptoms of this new flu because, as was later found, the virus was easily able to reach the cells of the digestive system. Moreover, the disease was resistant to two of the classic antivirals that were normally used, although it did respond to Tamiflu and Relenza.

Was it really swine flu?

The virus of the last flu pandemic was originally identified as coming from pigs, but we haven't yet managed to identify with absolute certainty the place where the pandemic started. The A(H1N1) virus has only been detected in pigs from two places but, in both cases, the animals were infected by a human and not the reverse. A Canadian who'd been in Mexico passed the virus into a herd of pigs when he returned home. The other case happened on a farm in Argentina.

As the OIE (World Organization for Animal Health) has noted, there's no proof demonstrating that pigs were somehow involved in the origin of the pandemic. Some scientists believe that birds could be the culprits, that the virus would have gone from pigs to birds some time earlier and birds ended up transmitting it to humans.

Mexican scientists and politicians claim they acted as fast as they could. In general, experts believe that the response of governments to the crisis was adequate. 'All possible means were tried in order to contain the pandemic and prevent contagion', says Dr Ana Fernández-Sesma. 'Notwithstanding, some countries overreacted and isolated noninfected people because of their nationality. The press was also somewhat alarmist in describing the epidemic as "lethal" and this caused a certain amount of panic.'[11]

The Mexican government recognized three separate outbreaks of the flu in its territory: in the capital, the centre and near the US border. It's said that the first person to be infected could have been a 5-year-old boy from La Gloria, a small town in the state of Veracruz, who caught the flu in March. Coincidentally, there are pig slaughterhouses nearby, belonging to an American company, but the A(N1H1) virus was never found, either in the animals or in the workers. Other theories suggest that there were earlier cases, among them a 6-month-old girl from San Luis Potosí in the heart of Mexico, who fell ill on 24 February. The first death of the epidemic was that of a 37-year-old diabetic woman named María, who was admitted to the Oaxaca hospital with flu-like symptoms. Although the first cases in Mexico were first seen in March 2009, it can't be claimed with any certainty that the epidemic began in the country.

In the first three weeks, the flu had caused eighteen deaths and about 1,000 people suspected of having it were admitted to hospital. Mortality among those infected was situated as being between 0.6 and 6 per cent, which, fortunately, were low figures by comparison with those for bird flu. Surprisingly, it affected young people but few among the elderly population. One of the explanations for this is that the virus bears some resemblance to others of the H1N1 type that had been responsible for the seasonal flu outbreaks some years earlier, so older people probably had some immunity against the new virus, thanks to the vaccines they had previously received.

11 See footnote 7.

Background: the 1976 flu

In 1976, there was an outbreak of swine flu, of an H1N1 variant, in the barracks of a US Army facility in New Jersey. There was only one death and, in the end, the flu didn't spread across the country. The US government immediately started a massive campaign in which President Gerald Ford aimed to vaccinate the whole population. Only a third received the vaccine and, unfortunately, the one that was used caused serious neurological problems in at least 500 people, 25 of whom died. One of the problems was the attempt to distribute it quickly before it had been subjected to the usual quality control tests. It must be said that the vaccines administered today are safer, and there are very few cases of adverse reactions.

The flu didn't take long to cross borders. By the end of April, seven cases had already been detected in the United States. Meanwhile, the Mexican authorities suspended classes in schools and universities. The WHO warned of the rapid spread of the epidemic and emphasized the fact that the virus came from animals, although it recognized that its low level of virulence meant that it wasn't very dangerous. The most serious cases were only seen at the beginning of the outbreak and in Mexico alone. In the rest of the world, it ran its course with milder symptoms and no deaths, but no one could really explain why.

The disease slowly spread through the United States. In New York, eight students from the neighbourhood of Queens, some of whom had recently travelled to Mexico, tested positive for the virus, but the clinical symptoms they presented weren't serious. After confirming about twenty cases of swine flu distributed around the country, from New York to Ohio,

Kansas, Texas and California, the US government announced that it was unable to control the virus because of its rapid spread. In response, the authorities decided to distribute a quarter of the national reserves of antiviral drugs to those states where the presence of the virus had been confirmed.

A lab virus?

As happened a decade later with SARS-CoV-2, it was at first suspected that the 2009 flu might have been artificial. Dr Adrian Gibbs, an eminent Australian virologist who worked in the development of Tamiflu, suggested that the A(H1N1) virus had been the result of a 'laboratory error'. In his view, some characteristics of the virus suggested that it had been produced in eggs which, as we've seen, is the usual way of cultivating viruses for study purposes. Dr Gibbs's theory was that the virus had appeared by accident in the process of producing a seasonal flu vaccine and, somehow, it escaped and infected pigs.

At the beginning of May 2009, the WHO announced that it would investigate all possibilities regarding the origin of the virus, including this one. A couple of weeks later, it was concluded that the studies demonstrated, without a shadow of doubt, that the virus was natural.

Meanwhile, in Mexico, many people believed that the government was exaggerating or inventing the whole story and refused to take measures. Another part of the population was convinced that the government was hiding the true extent of the epidemic. Some even claimed that the virus had been dumped by the United States. A similar reaction was seen later, with COVID-19, when some US politicians blamed China, saying that the coronavirus had emanated from one of its laboratories, while China counterattacked by asserting that SARS-CoV-2 had been imported by some US soldiers. These kinds of reaction seem inevitable, which is why it's so important to refute such stories as soon as possible with hard data, and to make sure that uncertainty doesn't give wings to rumour.

Television was abuzz with health recommendations (wash your hands well, don't shake hands, don't kiss anyone, and so on). Many people wore masks in the street, most of them useless for stopping a flu virus, but still selling for five times the normal price. The army started distributing approved masks gratis not long afterwards, even though experts insisted that they weren't very effective in stopping contagion, especially when worn in open spaces. Rather, they were recommended for the influenza patients and those caring for them. In churches, the 'kiss of peace' rite was suspended to avoid direct contact among parishioners, and football matches were played without spectators. Demonstrations were banned, as were public festivities, and cinemas were closed. Food couldn't be bought and consumed in shops or restaurants, where only takeaways were allowed.

No one escapes it

Viruses don't understand hierarchies. Some of the those whose names must be included among the thousands who caught swine flu are the son of Dr Anne Moscona, an influenza specialist at the Weill Medical College in New York; Cherie Blair, wife of the former British prime minister Tony Blair; Óscar Arias, then president of Costa Rica; and Rupert Grint, one of the stars of the Harry Potter films. All four recovered well and, in Grint's case, the ailment didn't even interrupt shooting an episode of the series.

The problem soon ceased to be confined to Mexico and the United States and became global. Cases were suspected in Colombia, Israel, France, Great Britain, New Zealand and Spain. In the latter case, eight people who had travelled to Mexico had symptoms of the flu. On 27 April, the first case in Spain, and also Europe, was finally confirmed, followed by two more cases in the United Kingdom. The virus had begun to sweep through the continent. The Spanish government and the European Union recommended against travelling to Mexico and the United States unless it was strictly necessary, although the WHO didn't deem it a priority measure at that point. In May, the Spanish Ministry of Defence quarantined barracks at the Hoyo de Manzanares military academy in Madrid after six soldiers showed flu-like symptoms and later tested positive for the A(H1N1) virus. All cases were mild, and everyone recovered.

The first person to die outside Mexico was a 2-year-old toddler. Born in Mexico, he was probably infected there, but he died in Texas twenty days after the first symptoms appeared. On the other side of the planet, in Hong Kong, a whole hotel was sealed and quarantined at the end of April when a guest coming from Mexico was found to have swine flu. This time, the infection was contained.

Meanwhile, stock exchanges around the world were reeling as oil prices plunged. At the same time, shares of the pharmaceutical companies GSK and Roche, which were producing antiviral treatments, were very much on the rise. The economic impact was also felt in tourism, of course, and in the food sector. Just as there was a significant drop in the consumption of chicken during the bird flu epidemic of 2004, so people stopped eating pork products in the pandemic of 2009. Some countries even banned imports of these items and set about implementing plans to sacrifice pigs in farms. These strategies, which have serious economic consequences, lack logical and scientific foundation and are totally useless anyway because the flu isn't transmitted by eating the flesh of infected animals.

Drugs and the race against time

Scientists immediately set to work to find a vaccine against the flu pandemic. Unlike COVID-19, in this case it was possible to take an already-existing vaccine and modify it slightly to adapt it to the new version of the virus. This greatly speeded up the process.

But the first bad news was that the virus reproduced less than normal in eggs, so it was difficult to work with. The dates for a possible vaccine that would be available to the public were initially set at between November 2009 and January 2010, a few months after the start of the pandemic (when, by contrast, the most optimistic forecasts in the case of COVID-19 estimate that the vaccine will take between twelve and eighteen months). Coordination among laboratories around the world was exemplary. As we've also seen later with COVID-19, scientists can work together and share data when necessary. Thanks to the joint work of experts, by 4 May there were more than 200 new entries with information about the genes of the H1N1 virus in the open-access database GenBank, where information about the human genome is also stored.

By the middle of July, it was announced that the production of the vaccine was between 25 and 50 per cent slower than originally envisaged because the virus wasn't generating the necessary quantity of haemagglutinin. The virus cultures were growing at a rate that was 30 per cent slower than those for the seasonal flu. The response was to go back to square one, with the consequent delay of several weeks. In Australia, the first tests of the vaccine began anyway at the end of July, using the samples that had been obtained, while the United States started testing at the beginning of August. By the end of the month, trials were being carried out with children and the first reactions seemed to indicate that the vaccine had no unanticipated side effects.

One of the tests that had to be done was mixing the vaccine against the flu pandemic with that for the seasonal flu to check whether the combination would create problems. The experts say that this doesn't represent any special risk because the flu vaccines presently being produced are very unlikely to cause complications and testing is practically a formality.

In May 2009, the pharmaceutical company Roche announced that it was donating 5.65 million packs of Tamiflu to the WHO so it could organize a 'rapid response' to the pandemic. The company's idea was to be able to offer the drug to developing countries at reduced prices. It also said that, if required, it could produce 110 million doses in five months, and up to 400 million treatments in a year. Apart from Roche, ten other pharmaceutical companies were producing generic drugs, so it was expected that the final count of antivirals would be greater.

Epidemic or pandemic?

Deciding whether or not an outbreak of infectious disease has become an epidemic or a pandemic depends only on its reach. Officially, the decision about when the classification of pandemic can be used (see box on p. 196) is made by the WHO, which is often under pressure to change a phase, or criticized when it's thought to have been too slow to act. With the swine flu in 2009, the alert started from Phase 3 of the

Flu pandemic phases of alert (according to the WHO)

1 No virus of those known to circulate among animals has infected humans.
2 It's confirmed that an animal flu virus has infected humans. Possible danger of a pandemic.
3 Small outbreaks in communities. There is no transmission of the virus between humans or only in a very small number of cases. The virus isn't yet capable of causing a pandemic.
4 Transmission among humans is common and verified. There's a high risk of a pandemic.
5 Transmission of the virus among humans is demonstrated in at least two countries in a geographic area defined by the WHO(*). A pandemic is imminent and fast action is needed to stop it spreading.
6 Beginning of a global pandemic. There's transmission among humans in a country of a region outside those defined in Phase 5.

(*) The areas are: Africa, the Americas, Europe, Southeast Asia, Eastern Mediterranean and Western Pacific

six possible stages as no significant transmission of the virus between humans had been seen at that point. On 27 April, it shifted to Phase 4, signifying that transmission among humans had been confirmed. Phase 5 began on 29 April when the risk of a pandemic was deemed imminent. A similar progression through the phases occurred with COVID-19 when the WHO resisted declaring a pandemic until it was already quite widespread. This is no trivial decision. Apart from questions of nomenclature, determining this status has an impact on the protocols that are recommended, which are different depending on whether there's a pandemic or not.

In spring 2009 it was evident that the new virus was spreading much faster than the seasonal flu but, loath to cause unnecessary panic, the WHO dithered about raising the alert level. Some experts believe that its response was too slow and that similar dilatoriness might create problems in case of a future pandemic caused by a more aggressive virus. In 2009, Dr Yi Gian, who discovered the SARS virus, said that Phase 5 should have been declared a couple of days earlier, and the fact that it wasn't contributed to the fact that the infection spread more quickly. A similar discussion took place with regard to COVID-19 and, once again, the WHO was blamed for not having acted fast enough and thereby facilitating the spread of the virus. Donald Trump even withdrew US funding from the UN as a way of objecting to what he said was an example of connivance with the Chinese government in soft-pedalling the outbreak.

With the A(H1N1) flu, there was even more reluctance to raise the alert to the last phase. Although the outbreak had met most of the conditions for being classified as Phase 6 by mid-May, it wasn't until 1 June 2009 that the WHO officially declared that the pandemic was under way. This was the first time in more than forty years that the much-feared Phase 6 had been reached, and it would take little more than a decade for a similar situation to appear.

By mid-July 2009, the benchmark figure of 100,000 people affected and 300 dead worldwide had been surpassed. The WHO recommended that counting each case should be discontinued, as the importance of the total number of infected people is negligible from the health point of view once a pandemic has been declared, and it only creates panic when newspapers start reporting it. Moreover, as happened later with COVID-19, some estimates suggest that the real number of infected people could be as much as twenty times greater than that for those cases that are diagnosed.

Thenceforth, laboratory tests for confirming the diagnosis were halted in many places, and everyone who presented with flu symptoms in the northern hemisphere was assumed to have caught the pandemic virus as the usual flu season had ended.

A change of hemispheres

At the end of June 2009, by which time more than 10,000 people in forty different countries had caught the pandemic influenza, with a death toll of about eighty, the disease was slowly moving into Asia. By the end of July, Japan had 300 cases and the first deaths had been recorded in India and southern Africa (where the victims were aged 14 and 22 respectively). Spain's first fatality, a 20-year-old Moroccan woman who had just given birth by caesarean, died at the end of June, and the tragedy was compounded when her baby died a few days later because of medical error. Some weeks later, it was discovered that pregnant women were especially sensitive to the pandemic influenza. The risk of their becoming seriously ill was four times higher, although they weren't infected any more easily than the rest of the population. It was therefore recommended to give Tamiflu to sick pregnant women as soon as possible, although some doctors were reluctant to prescribe it because of fear of harming the foetus.

Meanwhile, Russia blamed the United Kingdom for the cases that appeared within its borders and advised its citizens against travelling there (after having said the same thing about Spain some months earlier). Despite everything, the numbers of people infected and deaths were lower than believed at the beginning. Seeing that the consequences of the outbreak weren't too serious, the Mexican government had begun to allow restaurants and cafés to reopen in May, and also embarked on innovative strategies to revive tourism, for example offering free medical treatment to anyone spending a night in one of the country's hotels. This covered influenza or any other ailment and included medicines, transport and a stay in hospital.

As the United States was trying to get back to a normal existence, Australia was beginning to implement containment measures, since it was feared that the problem would move to other latitudes once the usual flu season began in the southern hemisphere. Contagion by the virus would be reactivated in the northern hemisphere with the coming of winter at the end of the year, so continued vigilance was all-important.

And indeed, the flu irrupted fast and strong in the southern hemisphere with the coming of winter. It's believed that there were 100,000 cases in Argentina, most of them in a matter of weeks after the onset of the cold weather and, by July, fifty-five deaths had been confirmed. It happened that the country had elections on 26 June, and some critics accused the government of hiding information in the run-up days, which would have helped the spread of the flu. It was later learned that a committee of experts had asked for a state of emergency to be decreed and had recommended that the elections be postponed (to avoid crowds), but the government refused. Shortly afterwards, a couple of lawyers privately sued the government on the grounds that it had endangered the health of citizens. The experts confirmed that even though the government knew the pandemic was coming, it had done nothing to prepare for it. It was said that the politicians were deliberately concealing data, for example by not counting sick people who went to private clinics in the total tally of those infected. Owing to the uncertainty, many Argentines travelled to Chile and Uruguay to buy antivirals, and the Brazilian and Bolivian governments were considering closing their borders to Argentines in order to prevent contagion.

Does it make sense to close schools?

There's no doubt that gatherings of children and young people aid the spread of any infectious disease, but the social problems occasioned by closing schools are greater than the benefits the measure can bring. If children must stay at home, many parents can't go to work, which could bring a whole country to a standstill.

After all, some experts say, the seasonal flu has high levels of contagion in schools, but this normally doesn't mean that classes must be suspended. The same debate has been aired during the COVID-19 pandemic. The schools finally closed when confinement began, although in some places they remained open throughout to cater to the children of essential personnel so that their parents could keep working. It's difficult to say whether closing schools in advance really has a significant impact in the number of cases.

In Chile, by contrast, there were more flu monitoring centres and, by the beginning of July, all large-scale events were cancelled. It also happened that the president, Michelle Bachelet, had trained as an epidemiologist, so she understood the importance of acting in time to stop contagion. Here, 99 per cent of the flu cases were from the A(H1N1) pandemic. But not everywhere was the same. In Australia, there was a mix of the two and, in South Africa, most cases were of the seasonal flu.

Coinciding with the coldest winter in a decade, that August Argentina was second to the United States in the worldwide death toll, with 261 fatalities. The hospitals were overwhelmed, and the government finally decided to close schools and cancel public events. The recommendation to stay at home meant a 60 per cent drop in sales at businesses in tourist destinations during the winter holidays. It was said that approximately 200,000 people were infected, but some observers believe that the real figure could very well be double that.

In Africa, the virus had been detected in nineteen countries by August and it was expected that this would be the continent that would have most problems as a result of the pandemic. Although thirteen African countries have WHO-approved centres for influenza studies, the difficulties involved in detecting outbreaks of the disease – and, above all, in distributing treatments and vaccines – prompted fears that the death toll would be much worse than in other places. Added to this was the problem of the continent's high percentage of AIDS cases, as it's been found that people infected with HIV are at greater risk of serious complications and death when they fall ill with flu. But perhaps the most important factor is that the rich countries monopolize all the drug production in advance. It was predicted that vaccines and antivirals wouldn't be produced fast enough to give them to all the people on the planet who needed them, and there was a good chance that Africa would be left without, while, in developed zones, most of the population would be covered. Only the WHO seemed concerned about this fact, while the other countries forgot about solidarity to focus on their own problems. Not a single government announced that it would allocate part of its scarce stocks to the neediest countries.

Prepare for the worst

Once the 2009 pandemic was declared, the UN Secretary-General met with representatives from the thirty drug companies that were producing influenza vaccines to be sure that there would be a ready response when A(H1N1) struck again in the northern hemisphere. The idea wasn't to stop producing vaccines against the seasonal flu but to start stepping up production of the swine flu vaccine as well. It was also stressed that production of enough antivirals should continue. Luckily, there aren't many cases of influenzas that can't be treated with Tamiflu. Resistant viruses have only been found in three countries, and all of those have responded to Relenza. There was nothing to suggest that this could become a serious problem but, just in case, some experts recommended keeping Tamiflu for the under-65s because it was predicted that it wouldn't reduce mortality in the over-65s, and using it in this group would probably contribute to the appearance of more resistance.

Meanwhile, in the United Kingdom, the number of influenza cases doubled in a few weeks although it was midsummer. There were about thirty deaths, a much lower figure that the usual number for seasonal flu but, even so, the government was beginning to think about delaying the start of the school year. As many as 65,000 deaths were predicted when the flu season arrived, though some observers considered that this estimate was greatly inflated. In the United States, 59 million cases of flu and 853,000 deaths were expected and, in Spain, about 8,000 fatalities were expected as the level of contagion at the time was very low: thirty-three people in every 100,000 caught the influenza (and, in August, the total number of cases was 26,000). In countries with more infections, the figure rose to sixty per 100,000.

In order to ensure that primary health centres wouldn't be overwhelmed, an innovative system was introduced in the United Kingdom. Instead of recommending that people should go to the doctor if they had influenza-like symptoms, they were asked to stay at home where, through a website or by phone, they could make their own diagnosis in a system similar to that used more recently for COVID-19. If it seemed that they were most probably infected, they were given a number by means of which they could go and collect a dose of Tamiflu at the nearest pharmacy. Although doctors were spared a considerable amount of work, the idea was soon criticized. There were fears that people would lie in the questionnaires so they could hoard a few doses of Tamiflu just in case, thus quickly exhausting the country's reserves. In the first few hours after the service began operating, the huge influx of queries blocked both online and phone consultations. Nevertheless, the experience was considered to be positive and a similar strategy was adopted in several countries during the COVID-19 pandemic.

In most of the northern hemisphere, the influenza pandemic seemed to be waning, but the alert continued until the end of summer as governments tried to get hold of as many doses of vaccines and antivirals as possible and started to make plans for a vaccination campaign. If everything turned out as expected and the virus didn't change, it was thought that, by autumn, about 10 per cent of the Spanish population, for example, could be infected but that 95 per cent of cases would be mild. Spain ordered from the companies Novartis and GSK enough units of the A(H1N1) vaccine to protect up to 40 per cent of its citizens, with the idea of vaccinating all under-15s and essential workers, a total of 18 million doses at a cost of around €266 million. In other developed countries, the orders covered up to 60 per cent of the population (see box on p. 204).

Who should be given the vaccine?

The first pandemic of the century made it clear that, in case of emergency, there aren't enough vaccines for everyone. If the choice must be made, who is given priority for receiving the vaccine? The logical answer would be people at risk, especially children, pregnant women and the elderly, as well as firemen, transport drivers, teachers, health workers and so on. But every country has its own plans in these situations about the doses of vaccines to which it has access. And they also differ depending on which virus causes the pandemic.

A study published in *Science* at the end of August 2009 stated that the best strategy for stopping the flu pandemic at the time was to vaccinate all school-age children and their parents, because schools were the main point of transmission of the virus. This disputed the original plan of vaccinating the under-5s and over-50s.

In Spain, the idea was to vaccinate all under-14s and up to 40 per cent of the population. Initially, the United States wanted to vaccinate most of the under-25s and over-64s (some 160 million people, at least), and the rest if enough doses were available. Greece wanted to vaccinate everyone, including illegal immigrants, with the 24 million doses it expected to have ready. This was also Holland's plan. The United Kingdom counted on being able to vaccinate 50 per cent of the population, while the figure in France was up to 70 per cent. Canada envisaged vaccinating 75 per cent of its population, bearing in mind the fact that two doses of the vaccine were needed if it was to be effective. Fortunately, these vaccines were not needed in the end.

All these predictions depended on whether enough doses could be produced at the expected rate. As I noted above, the virus couldn't be cultivated as effectively as hoped in the beginning, which seriously affected the availability of the vaccine. As a result, at the end of August, it was calculated that the United States would only receive, in mid-November, 45 million out of the 120 million doses that were initially ordered. Other countries had the same problems. It was calculated that the pandemic might have affected 30 per cent of the world's population but, in the end, the real number would be 2–5 per cent infected, of whom only 0.4 per cent would die. Most of the dead would be people with immune deficiency or other prior health problems. In fact, the final numbers weren't too far from the predictions: 11–21 per cent of people were infected, but mortality was lower than envisaged, at around 0.03 per cent (between 150,000 and 575,000 dead).

The consequences of the pandemic

In the end, the impact of the 2009 pandemic wasn't much worse than that of a seasonal flu, despite its faster propagation and the panic in the early stages. The reasons for alarm disappeared once the minimum appropriate measures had been taken, at least in the developed countries. However, in some countries, the response of citizens to the whole experience, and notably to the special treatment given to the pandemic by the press, and the sometimes confused messages from political leaders, was almost unanimously negative. In Spain, for example, a survey in early September 2009 indicated that 87 per cent of respondents believed that the social anxiety over the A(H1N1) influenza was an over-reaction. Many videos and letters, some posted by doctors, were circulating online, criticizing the performance of the authorities and accusing the pharmaceutical companies of deliberately whipping up fear so they could sell more drugs.

This perception could have had an influence in holding back preparations for a possible future pandemic. So, when COVID-19 struck, it was at a time when the great majority of countries didn't have contingency plans designed to deal with a crisis of this kind. One could say, then, that the 2009 influenza crisis would have hampered any attempt to be ready for the next pandemic because of this climate of mistrust, which arose from the fact that many people believed the response in 2009 was overblown. It's important to remember that, when a new virus appears, we can't predict how aggressive it will be. Instead of being thankful that the A(H1N1) influenza pandemic wasn't as serious as feared, and using this experience as a foundation for future readiness, preventive actions were hampered, as if in some postmodern version of the boy who cried wolf. If we'd understood that the 2009 influenza pandemic was a warning of worse diseases that could hit us in future, COVID-19 wouldn't have caused such an upheaval because we would have been ready to nip it in the bud.

Now, it will be important to learn from our mistakes and be better prepared for next time. We've seen what can happen when a virus brings on a pandemic that doesn't go away by itself, and the point to which it can rock the foundations of the world order, and we've probably finally learned that it can't be taken lightly. We don't know when the next pandemic will strike or what virus will cause it, but it could be equally as serious or worse than (let's hope not!) COVID-19. It's therefore essential to have plans of action ready in case we ever find ourselves faced with a worst-case scenario because, in such serious situations, not reacting promptly enough means the loss of thousands of lives.

Beyond its seasonal version, influenza continues to be a major danger. The possibility of a new drastic pandemic with an 'improved' version of the A(H1N1) virus is still present. This is what happened with the bird flu virus H5N1: nobody can guarantee that these viruses will keep acting in future in the same way they've done so far. Genetic studies have demonstrated that the virus of the influenza pandemic didn't have a variant of the PB1-F2 protein, which is associated, precisely, with high levels of virulence, and this is why mortality was so low. The chances that A(H1N1) will disappear by itself are slim. It is probable, then, that it will remain with us, and we will never know whether it will evolve to become more aggressive or stay as it is for evermore. It has therefore joined the list of dangerous viruses that could spread again if given the right conditions.

To sum up what I've said in this chapter, influenza will continue to be a major health problem at the global level for as long as there's no universal vaccine because of the mortality rates caused by its seasonal version, not to mention the risk of a pandemic set off by a sufficiently aggressive form of the virus. In the words of Dr Fernández-Sesma: 'It'd be better if we never stopped fearing influenza because it could come back in a more virulent form at any time. We still need to get all the governments to abide by the international WHO norms and ensure that the poorer countries have fast access to drugs and vaccines at no extra cost.'[12]

12   See footnote 7 on p. 154.

8

AIDS

Some people believe that AIDS, or Acquired Immunodeficiency Syndrome, may be the worst plague that has ever afflicted humanity. On the global scale, it's estimated that 38 million people were infected, 68 per cent in sub-Saharan Africa and 18 per cent in Southeast Asia, with an increase of 2.5 million infections every year. Since 2002, AIDS has been the main cause of death by infectious disease in Africa. More than 60 million people are thought to have been infected, some 25 million have died since the beginning of the pandemic and the numbers aren't standing still: 770,000 people died because of AIDS in 2018, and the figures probably won't be going down much as there are more than 1.5 million new infections every year. Between 2008 and 2010, about 42 million children lost one or both parents to AIDS, especially in sub-Saharan Africa.

Despite the gravity of these data, there's a false perception in the developed countries that the disease no longer represents a danger. This means that efforts to bolster prevention strategies often fail, especially as they have little impact on people at risk. For example, although new cases of AIDS in Southern Europe have been falling steadily since the beginning of the century, genetic studies have placed Spain on the list of the chief AIDS 'exporters' among the European countries, together with Greece, Portugal and Serbia. The reason

Myth and reality: how is AIDS spread?

There are many wrong ideas about how AIDS is transmitted. In a 2009 survey in Spain, 20 per cent of the respondents believed that infected people had to be isolated or that their names should be published on a list; 34 per cent were convinced that the disease could be caused by a mosquito bite, while between 30 and 40 per cent confessed they would feel uncomfortable if they knew that there was an infected person in the place where they shopped, or at their children's school, to the point that they would even demand that the person be moved.

But HIV is only acquired through sexual contact (the virus is found in all male and female fluids involved in intercourse), by injection of blood (transfusions or a used syringe) or when it's passed from mother to child (during birth or in her milk). It's been found that a person with a venereal disease (herpes, gonorrhoea or syphilis) is more susceptible to being infected with AIDS through sexual contact.

Otherwise, no other secretion (saliva, sweat, etc.) has been found to have the virus in sufficient quantities to be contagious. Moreover, unlike the flu virus, HIV can't survive well outside the human body. It's recently been found that it can be passed on in some cultures where the mother masticates food before giving it to her children, but this seems to be due to the presence of blood, so saliva isn't to blame.

is that tourists travelling to these places are often infected after unprotected sex and they then spread the disease in their countries of origin. The experts agree that the AIDS pandemic is by no means under control and that it's impossible to predict how long it will last.

Another multifaceted virus

One of the reasons why AIDS is such a difficult disease to beat is the extraordinary changeability of the virus responsible, HIV (human immunodeficiency virus). Two forms exist that infect humans, HIV-1 and HIV-2. The former is more aggressive, while the latter is only found in some parts of West Africa. There are three main types of HIV-1 (called M, N and O), and a new one (called P) was discovered in the summer of 2009 in a 62-year-old woman from Cameroon.

There are at least a million different versions of HIV scattered around the world. With viruses of the same type there can be variations of up to 20 per cent in the genome and, in the case of the proteins that form the cover of the virus (normally those used to make vaccines), the differences can be as great as 38 per cent. Furthermore, within one infected person, the virus will keep evolving until, after a time, there are thousands upon thousands of variants. It's easy to understand, therefore, that finding the proper tools that will enable us to stop all these changing forms from appearing presents a major logistical problem.

The African sickness

Surprising as it may seem, the AIDS virus started infecting humans more than a century ago. Both HIV-1 and HIV-2 come from a family of viruses (the simian immunodeficiency virus or SIV) that attack monkeys in the central and western zones of Africa. Chimpanzees are possibly the primates in which the pandemic began, and it seems likely that HIV type M came to humans through an ape that infected just one person, most probably in the south of Cameroon in the early years of the twentieth century. It's also thought that type P could be the only variant that comes from gorillas.

Until recently, it was supposed that chimpanzees with SIV in their blood didn't fall ill. Humans and macaques, however, suffer from a severe autoimmune syndrome when infected by the corresponding viruses. One theory attempting to explain these differences between species of primates postulated that, in humans and macaques, the immune system responds more aggressively to the infection, thus increasing the destruction of cells and lowering defences. But eventually scientists discovered chimpanzees in which SIV had indeed brought on the disease.

Rumours

It's said that, in the early days of the pandemic, the Russian government spread the tale, through a British journalist, that the US Army had created the virus in a laboratory and had unleashed it on Africa. American scientists hastened to respond to the articles saying that HIV was too complex and that they didn't even understand how it worked. There was no laboratory in the world that would be capable of making it. With time, it's been confirmed that the true origins of the pandemic have nothing to do with humans.

It's not known exactly how the virus went from monkey to man, or why it wasn't until many years later that there was such a dramatic hike in the number of infections. One theory suggests that the virus needs a considerable concentration of people in order to propagate effectively. At first, this wouldn't have been possible in Africa, where people were widely dispersed until the development of modern cities. It's believed that propagation spread out from the city of Leopoldville (now Kinshasa), the biggest in the area in the early years of the twentieth century, and capital of what is now the Democratic Republic of the Congo. AIDS would then be a pandemic typical of our times, spurred on by the arrival of progress in an endemic zone.

Analysis of the oldest conserved samples infected with HIV, dating from 1959 and 1960, suggests that the pandemic among humans would have begun in the early decades of the twentieth century, with just a few infected individuals. Transmission would have been progressing exponentially and, by the 1960s, there must have been several thousand infected people, all of them still in central Africa. It's believed that the virus travelled to Haiti in around 1966 and, in 1969, entered the United States thanks to immigration from the island. But the AIDS pandemic didn't become evident until 1981, when a large cluster of unusual ailments especially affecting homosexuals – among them pneumonia brought on by the fungus *Pneumocystis*, and a very rare

The myth of 'patient zero'

It's said that AIDS spread rapidly among homosexuals in the early 1980s because of a so-called 'patient zero', an especially promiscuous flight attendant who had sex with at least forty of the first individuals with AIDS to be detected outside Africa and the Caribbean. This, however, is difficult to confirm.

skin cancer called Kaposi's sarcoma – began to appear in the United States. Initially, called GRID (gay-related immuno-deficiency), the disease spread quickly among the four at-risk populations, then called the 4H Club: homosexuals, heroin addicts, haemophiliacs and Haitians.

A scientists' squabble

In 1983, the French virologists Luc Montagnier and Françoise Barré-Sinoussi announced that they had discovered a virus that might be the cause of the strange epidemic. The following year, their most direct rival, the American researcher Robert Gallo, published a series of four articles in the prestigious journal *Science* claiming that he had isolated a new virus in several patients, that it was the cause of AIDS and was of the HTLV family. He also noted that, some years earlier, his laboratory had found that these viruses induce leukaemia. He had therefore decided to call the new virus HTLV-III. But the viruses found in France and the United States turned out to be the same, and it slowly emerged that their similarities with the HTLV viruses were, in fact, minimal. Hence, a committee of experts eventually decided to call the discovery HIV, despite Gallo's vehement opposition.

The wrangle among scientists over who discovered HIV kept escalating. The problem wasn't only a matter of who got the glory; also at stake was an immense amount of money that would be generated by tests to detect the virus. France and the United States wanted this for themselves, and pressure from politicians in both countries became apparent.

It took mediation by the countries' respective presidents, Ronald Reagan and Jacques Chirac, to get the two groups of scientists to settle their differences in 1987. They agreed to share the honours for the discovery, which they announced with the publication of a joint article in *Nature*. In it, they recognized that Gallo had declared in a congress that a retrovirus was responsible for AIDS some months before Montagnier had published his article identifying it. With this Solomonic gesture, they also agreed to share the economic proceeds as each country would get an equal part of the possible benefits.

The controversy was far from over. In 1989, an article published in the *Chicago Tribune* denounced the fact that the virus Gallo had supposedly isolated was exactly the same as the one Montagnier and Barré-Sinoussi had identified a year earlier. The samples studied in Gallo's laboratory were simply the ones that the French scientists had sent him in a gesture of good will, which was the usual practice among scientists. So, Gallo hadn't discovered any new virus at all and, therefore, deserved none of the glory.

So, who discovered HIV?

Once the dust settled after the initial row, the consensus has been that Montagnier and Barré-Sinoussi isolated the virus, but it was Gallo who first established experimentally that HIV causes AIDS. Moreover, he managed to cultivate it in the laboratory and to design a scientific method for detecting it.

An investigation was immediately launched to ascertain whether this was, in fact, a case of scientific fraud. When it concluded in 1993, Gallo had been able to demonstrate that the 'errors' in his studies were unintentional as his own samples had accidentally been contaminated by the French virus. We will probably never know whether Gallo deliberately resorted to skulduggery to eclipse the role of Montagnier and his team. However, since it was clear that Gallo had used Montagnier's virus in his experiments, the US government was sued by the French government and had to cede a share in the royalties it collected for sales of blood tests by its licensees.

The Nobel of discord

Despite the official version of the events, when half the 2008 Nobel Prize in Medicine was awarded to the discoverers of HIV, only Luc Montagnier and Françoise Barré-Sinoussi received gold medals. The prize committee completely dismissed Gallo's role. The other half of the prize went to a different field: the discovery of the link between HPV infection and cervical cancer.

Montagnier at once declared that he wished Gallo had been included in the prize because he deserved it as much as he and Barré-Sinoussi did. Numerous letters of support for Gallo, deploring the error of judgement made by the Swedish Academy, were published in specialist journals, among them one in *Science* signed by more than 100 scientists, some of them leading experts in the field. Gallo elegantly confessed that he was disappointed to have been overlooked but, nevertheless, congratulated his colleagues.

Besides his contributions in the area of HIV, in the 1970s Robert Gallo took part in the first discoveries of cancer-related viruses, and also of IL-2, a key protein in the immune system. He has received more than eighty prizes, among them America's most prestigious mark of recognition for biomedical research, the Lasker award, which is often a precursor to a Nobel prize. Indeed, he received two Lasker awards – the only person to have achieved this feat. But, apart from his scientific merits, he's always had the reputation of being a controversial figure. Some of his detractors have accused him of delaying for a year introduction into the United States of a method for detecting the virus developed by the French scientists, and that, as a result, many people were infected by HIV because of contaminated blood from infected donors. Others claim that he obstructed HIV research as much as he could in the early days, even going so far as to publish false data in order to mislead the competition. In the book *And the Band Played On: Politics, People, and the AIDS Epidemic* (by journalist Randy Shilts), Gallo is described as being obsessed with his own reputation and engaging in political manipulation to discredit his rivals. Scientists who have worked with him anonymously describe him as self-seeking and unscrupulous, and his laboratory as a 'den of thieves', like a medieval fiefdom where, it was also rumoured, he had at least one lover. It was said, too, that he once bragged that he liked to contract foreign scientists because, if they didn't do what he wanted, he could get them deported. Moreover, he was accused of stealing confidential ideas, appropriating other people's discoveries and sabotaging samples so that colleagues couldn't advance with their research. To cap it all, some sources even say he had a penchant for making middle-of-the-night prank phone calls to his rivals.

How much of these stories is true and how much is legend, only those involved will know. That Gallo would seem to have earned his enemies, for whatever reason, is demonstrated not only by the fact that he didn't get a Nobel prize but he was also denied – on six occasions – the most important scientific honour of the United States, which is to say membership of the National Academy of Sciences.

The silent infection

In addition to its variability, HIV has another powerful weapon: its ability to infect an important type of immune system cell (a white blood cell known as a lymphocyte, and specifically, those with a receptor called CD4) and remain there in a 'latent' state. Unnoticed, it lies in wait, without reproducing or killing the cell it has invaded, so it can't be destroyed by any known drug or by our own defences.

Some years after the original infection, the latent virus will reactivate and start to divide, for reasons that still aren't totally clear. This ends up killing the CD4 lymphocytes, thus causing the cell count to plummet, as blood tests show, and leading to the well-known drop in defences. This is why the full-blown disease, AIDS, develops long after the original HIV infection.

Another fact that contributes enormously to the pandemic is that, during this stealthy latent period, infected people, often unaware of having the virus in their bloodstream and

Closing borders

In 1987, the United States adopted a much-criticized measure – banning entry to the country of all HIV-positive foreigners – in an attempt to stop the spread of AIDS. People who wanted to cross the border had to fill in a form that included the question about AIDS.

Subsequent studies have shown that the measure was of no real use and, in 2008, President George W. Bush signed a counter-order to revoke the law. But other countries still have similar measures, among them China, the United Arab Emirates and South Korea.

not taking proper precautions, can pass it on to many others. The WHO calculates that 80 per cent of people who are infected with HIV don't know they have it. The first sign of contagion can be confused with a cold. Two or three weeks after HIV enters the body, the virus steps up its reproduction, which gives flu-like symptoms, but they quickly disappear. A few months later, there's a balance between the virus and immune cells which, over the years, will be lost when it tips in favour of the virus.

In the visible phase of the disease, as soon as the HIV virus has destroyed enough immune cells, people who've contracted it start to suffer serious, unexpected secondary infections. For example, bacteria that normally harmoniously coexist with us start attacking the body when the immune system is no longer able to control them. The digestive tract is one of the places where the loss of defences is fastest and most devastating, which is why many infections are seen in this area. Pneumonia (especially a type caused by the fungus *Pneumocystis*, rarely seen outside cases of AIDS) and tuberculosis are also common. The frequency of cancers, in particular lymphomas, also increases. Since no organ escapes the effects of this implacable demolition of the immune system, there can be many final causes of death.

It's known that men and women respond differently to the virus, although it's not really understood why. Women tend to have lower levels than men of HIV in their blood, yet their progression to AIDS is faster. This might be due to the fact that a woman's immune system is more strongly activated when it detects the virus, which means that the lymphocytes are destroyed more rapidly. And it's thought that the reason for this could be hormonal.

Necessary swift diagnosis

Diagnosing an HIV infection is done by means of the ELISA technique, which detects the antibodies present in the serum generated by the human body against the virus. Hence, people infected by it are called *seropositive*. If this is later confirmed using another technique called Western blot, the error rates in the diagnosis are less than 0.003 per cent. There are also simpler and faster procedures, but they are not so sensitive and less specific than ELISA. Nevertheless, they are more useful in developing countries where there's frequently no access to the equipment needed to carry out more precise tests.

Many countries have programmes under way for offering a free HIV diagnosis for adults. Fast tests, taking fifteen minutes, tend to be used, and, if the result is positive, it's recommended that the person seek confirmation by other more accurate means. The advantage of quick methods is that they don't require special knowledge and can be used anywhere, which makes them ideal for diagnosis in developing countries.

Being able to extend early diagnosis to the greater part of the globe is one of the foremost objectives in plans to prevent transmission of the disease. The American College of Physicians went so far as to propose that absolutely everyone over the age of 13 should have the test every year. In 2006, US government experts recommended introducing a system in which everyone between the ages of 13 and 64 attending a health centre in the country should routinely have the AIDS test, unless the person expressly asked not to have it. The measure wasn't implemented because some states require written consent for any test carried out, and because the insurance companies refused to bear the costs.

According to WHO estimates, such initiatives could cut new infections by up to 95 per cent in less than a decade if accompanied by prevention measures and immediate anti-retroviral treatment for people who test positive. If these steps were taken, the AIDS pandemic could probably be stopped in fifty years. The problem is that this would be expensive (up to $3,400 million per year) and, in any case, such initiatives demonstrate the importance of social involvement and fieldwork in making the medical advances available to everyone, whether in the form of diagnosis or treatment. Eradication of diseases like AIDS, which affect the more impoverished social groups, requires the involvement of governments, foundations and NGOs. Science alone isn't enough. Social activism in the case of AIDS has been an asset since the beginning of the pandemic and has contributed significantly to the success of the measures of containment that are presently being applied.

A miraculous treatment ... that doesn't cure

At present, there's no cure for AIDS. No known medicine can eliminate HIV from an infected person. Yet we've managed to find an acceptable solution: a series of drugs called *antiretrovirals*, which prevent HIV from reproducing and keep it under control.

Antiretrovirals have dramatically reduced mortality. The first to be discovered, in 1987, was zidovudine (ZDV), also known as azidothymidine (AZT), but treatment with a single drug meant that the virus quickly developed resistance. It wasn't until 1995 that a new class of antiretrovirals, protease inhibitors, appeared, and more than two drugs were combined in the treatment. Complex mathematical models made it possible to predict that a three-drug cocktail would be the most effective approach, and this was demonstrated to be the case in 1996. HIV is particularly sensitive to these drugs, which keep virus levels in the blood to below minimum levels for a long time and, some say, maybe for life. This represented an important qualitative change and the treatment has been improving ever since. At present, twenty-five antiretroviral drugs, of seven different types, have been approved for combating HIV. Instead of being an inescapable death sentence, as it was in the early days, AIDS has become a chronic illness.

Strange bedfellows

The peculiarities of treating AIDS have led to some very unusual alliances being forged between pharmaceutical companies. While Roche announced that it was ceasing its AIDS research at the beginning of 2009, the giants GSK and Pfizer merged their divisions researching new medication. Together, these two companies produce 20 per cent of all antiretrovirals. This merger has a precedent. For some years now, Gilead Sciences and BSM have been selling a combination of drugs, called Atripla, which is now one of the most commonly used.

The current treatment regime is called HAART (highly active antiretroviral therapy) and consists of at least three drugs of a minimum of two types. This treatment is especially effective in preventing transmission from mother to child if given during pregnancy and the baby's first six months. The possibility of infection then drops from 30 per cent to only 2 per cent. One of the obstacles is the high cost of the treatment, which is lifelong. As a result, it doesn't reach people living in the more disadvantaged countries, which are precisely those with most cases. Unsurprisingly, the highest numbers of children with AIDS are found in sub-Saharan Africa, while in countries like the United States, AIDS-related child mortality has fallen by 90 per cent in the last twenty years.

Left untreated, AIDS kills, on average, nine months after the first symptoms appear (about twelve years after infection). Antiretrovirals can prolong this period almost indefinitely. If someone is infected at about 20 years of age and starts taking antiretrovirals before the immune cell count falls too low, his or her life expectancy could be around 63 years (twenty years less than normal). However, up to 50 per cent of patients can't benefit from the treatment because of intolerance, side effects of the drugs or because they've been infected with a resistant type of HIV.

More options

New and better antiretrovirals that attack the virus's weak points are constantly being produced. For example, Raltegravir, which was approved for use in the United States in 2007, and was already being used in Australia, finally came to Europe in 2008. The first of a new class of antiretrovirals called integrase inhibitors, it has proved to be effective in patients showing resistance. The first clinical trial, which lasted two years and was made public in the summer of 2009, demonstrated very potent anti-HIV activity and few secondary effects in the short term.

An added difficulty is deciding when the HAART treatment should begin. Originally, it was delayed for as long as possible to avoid secondary effects. Recent studies, however, recommend starting early on. The sign for starting antiretroviral treatment is when the CD4 lymphocytes drop below a minimum level (350 cells per cubic millilitre of blood, when the normal figure is 1,200). If treatment is given earlier, when the cells are still at a level of above 500 per cubic millilitre, the chances of AIDS not appearing are almost certainly better. Some people believe that if the infection is dealt with early enough, and the treatment is sufficiently aggressive, it might even be possible to eliminate the virus from the organism. But the more time that goes by, the harder this would be to achieve.

In line with these principles, a preventive measure called PrEP (pre-exposure prophylaxis) was produced with the idea of administering drugs against the virus as a preventive measure to people who are not yet infected but are members of an at-risk population. A combination of two or three of the classic antiretrovirals (the best known, perhaps, being Truvada, which is produced by Gilead) is given, and it's believed that the protection offered by this treatment is almost 100 per cent. Although it's so useful, PrEP is only available in some countries and its price is prohibitive in the zones where it would be most needed.

Side effects

Some patients have been receiving the HAART treatment for decades, thus keeping the infection under control. Since antiretrovirals have been known for a relatively short time, we still don't know the long-term consequences of continually taking such aggressive drugs, or whether their side effects will be permanent. However, other kinds of treatment, like those normally administered with PrEP, don't seem to have significant side effects.

It's known, for instance, that all these drugs affect lipid levels (cholesterol, triglycerides), and it has been found recently that there are also rising instances of heart and liver diseases, as well as diabetes, among HIV-positive people who have been receiving treatment for a long time, though there is as yet no evidence that these phenomena are related. There has also been an increase in cancers, especially of the liver, lungs and anus, as well as melanomas and Hodgkin lymphoma, none of which are, in principle, related to the virus (as Kaposi sarcoma and non-Hodgkin lymphoma certainly are). We still don't know the reason for these increases.

Apart from these side effects, there are others which, while they may be less serious, can still significantly affect the patient's quality of life. One example is lipodystrophy, an abnormal distribution of fat in the body, which is seen in almost half the people receiving HAART treatment. Patients lose fat in the face and extremities and accumulate it in the torso, to the point of considerable deformity. With the disappearance of fat from the face, the cheeks become sunken, leaving HIV-positive people with the typical 'skull-like' appearance associated with the infection, thus betraying their condition and perhaps resulting in social stigmatization. It is believed that these are direct side effects of antiretroviral activity, perhaps combined with that of the virus itself.

Research groups like those of Dr Marta Giralt and Dr Francesc Villarroya at the University of Barcelona are studying the molecular bases of these fatty tissue disorders in the hope of finding the cause and coming up with a possible treatment. Thanks to their research and that of other leading groups around the world, it's now known that the appearance of these problems can be prevented up to a point by avoiding certain combinations of antiretroviral drugs. 'When deciding a treatment, it's important to be able to analyse the potential of the different antiretroviral drugs to affect the lipid metabolism', says Dr Giralt. 'We carry out studies with fat cells in the laboratory in order to determine the least toxic combinations for patients. These studies aiming at ascertaining the mechanisms that cause lipodystrophy can also help us to understand fat-related diseases, for example those associated with obesity.'[13]

As long as no solutions are found at the pharmaceutical level, surgery is, for the moment, the best treatment option. The group led by Dr Joan Fontdevila, head of the Plastic Surgery Service at Hospital Clínic, Barcelona, is carrying out pioneering work on the complex surgical technique used in these cases. The problem is solved by injecting into the cheeks some kind of synthetic tissue or, better still, fat taken from the patient's own abdomen or breast. 'Normalizing the patient's appearance goes beyond frivolous cosmetic retouching', Joan Fontdevila observes. 'It's equally or more important than the antiretroviral treatment. Drugs can control the disease, and reconstructive surgery pre-empts the appearance of psychological disorders associated with social rejection.' This can lead to mental problems like anxiety or depression, which, in turn, affect how conscientiously patients continue with their antiretroviral treatment. 'The repercussions of this disorder are important in the patient's family and working life', Fontdevila says. 'One treatment shouldn't be contemplated without the other.'[14] Some countries, like Spain, the United Kingdom and France, have understood that this is true and now offer surgery to patients with lipodystrophy if they should need it.

13 From an interview by the author with Marta Giralt [translation: JW].
14 From an interview by the author with Joan Fontdevila [translation: JW].

The virus becomes more dangerous

It is difficult to find a virus that is insensitive to all the anti-retrovirals presently being used, but it's also true that HIV is starting to develop resistance to some of them. It's calculated that between 5 and 15 per cent of new infections are caused by viruses showing some kind of resistance. At present, new systems of diagnosis are being developed for better detection of these viruses and in order to ascertain the point to which they are a health risk.

In addition to resistance, HIV infections are markedly more aggressive today than they were twenty years ago. In other words, by the time HIV-positive people go to hospital and discover they have the virus, their immune cell count is already lower. This might be explained by increased virulence in the presently circulating forms of HIV. In fact, in

The false 'superbug'

In 2005, newspapers reported the case of a homosexual man in New York who was found to have a type of HIV that was resistant to all known drugs. Moreover, it seemed that it could trigger AIDS only a few months after infection, and not years later, as is the usual pattern. The frightening, unstoppable 'superbug' epidemic (as the American press called it) was the talk of the town.

After several genetic studies had been carried out, it was found that the supposed superbug was neither new nor more aggressive than other types. The reason the patient developed AIDS so quickly was probably due to other facts (for example, promiscuity, which might have enabled infection by a more aggressive strain; or drug use, which debilitates defences).

recent years, cases of what's been called fulminating AIDS have begun to appear among patients who develop immunodeficiency very shortly after becoming infected. If they aren't treated in time, death is imminent. In Europe, the first cases of fulminating AIDS were seen in the early 2000s. It's believed that this form of AIDS appeared as a result of a combination of these more potent viruses and an already weakened immune system. Fortunately, the aggressive variants are infrequent and aren't easily transmitted between people. Hence, there doesn't seem to be any imminent danger at the global level, although isolated cases will still appear.

Treatments for the future

HAART won't be an effective long-term solution to AIDS because, owing to its characteristics, it isn't accessible to everyone who needs it. In 2006, the WHO had set the goal of everyone having access to treatment before 2010, but this was soon seen to be optimistic and, even today, it's an aim that's far from being achieved. One of the problems is economic. In order to treat all infected people, an investment in drugs amounting to $90,000 million would need to be made (as the cost of the treatment can come close to $23,000 per person per year). It's therefore necessary to keep researching in order to find better drugs than HAART, and ways to eliminate the virus so it will no longer be necessary to continue the treatment forever.

The experimental treatment with the most encouraging results to date is bone marrow transplant. As sometimes happens, the discovery was more or less accidental. A 42-year-old patient with leukaemia, who was also HIV-positive, was to receive bone marrow stem cell treatment, one of the most promising options for the type of cancer he had. But Dr Gero Hütter, the haematologist who was treating him, had an idea. Since he was to receive cells from a donor, why not look for one with genetic resistance to AIDS? It's known that a small proportion of people aren't easily infected with HIV, although the reason for this isn't very clear. One thing that's thought to be a determinant is a certain variation in the CCR5 gene, which is found in 1 per cent of Europeans. CCR5 is one of the receptors on the surface of immune cells that HIV enters, but the virus doesn't easily recognize receptors with this variation and thus can't get into the cells. Dr Hütter found such a person in the databases, from among eighty who were genetically compatible with his patient. The transplant was a great success. When the story came to light in November 2008, two years after the patient had received the stem cells, there was no detectable trace of HIV in his blood even though he wasn't being treated for it. And there was no sign of leukaemia either. In March 2019, it was announced that a second case, in the United Kingdom, involved an HIV-positive patient with Hodgkin lymphoma who had no trace of the virus a year and a half after a bone marrow transplant similar to that used to treat Hütter's patient. Sadly, he died of his cancer in 2020.

For the moment, these are isolated cases. Furthermore, in the second case, follow-up has been too brief to be sure that the virus won't reappear. More experiments will be needed to see whether bone marrow stem cells can really be an effective treatment. The main problem is that the transplant is a risky procedure with possible secondary effects that are much more serious than those of antiretrovirals. So, it's not recommendable in most cases, which is why it's only been tried so far when it was necessary to treat HIV-positive patients who also have leukaemia. It's still necessary to find out more about the factors that determine resistance to HIV in order to select better donors, but this is a technique that could be useful in future, at least with certain patients.

It would be ideal, of course, to achieve the same effect without the associated risks. Pfizer is marketing in the United States and Europe a CCR5 inhibitor drug called Maraviroc, and other pharmaceutical companies are working along similar lines. Maraviroc could be quite effective if given with other drugs. Following these principles, tests are being done with gene therapy techniques. The idea is to take cells from the patient's immune system, genetically modify them in the laboratory (for example by eliminating the CCR5 gene that makes a person susceptible to being infected by HIV), and then to inject them back. But, for the moment, little is known about the effectiveness of these methods.

Other initiatives in the experimental phases include converting stem cells into immune cells to replace those of patients. Another attempt is to apply the RNA interference (RNAi) technique to AIDS treatment. The mechanism is based on small fragments of RNA that are capable of specifically inhibiting the functions of a gene. In the case of AIDS, the idea is to use RNAi to suppress replication of the virus. For example, one aim is to apply RNAi to vagina cells and thus prevent the entry of HIV.

Finally, another promising field is that of virus 'reactivators'. As I said, one of the characteristics of HIV is its ability to stay tucked away inside cells in such a way that drugs can't destroy it. Some recently discovered substances can force HIV out of its latency and get it to start replicating again, thus making it susceptible to antiretrovirals once more. The combination of reactivators and antiretrovirals might make it possible to 'cleanse' the body of the virus more effectively and, in theory, even eliminate it completely. The first reactivator to be discovered, HMBA, had too many side effects.

Also studied is another one called SAHA, which could be a less toxic alternative. And a further possibility is to combine HAART with certain chemotherapy treatments similar to those used with cancer, also with the aim of eliminating the dormant viruses.

At a scientific conference in the summer of 2020, it was announced that HIV had been eliminated from a 36-year-old Brazilian man who had tested positive. Known as the 'São Paulo Patient', he had received intensive antiretroviral therapy paired with nicotinamide, a potential reactivator of the virus, for forty-eight weeks, followed by three years of the usual therapy. After this, his treatment had been interrupted and, surprisingly, the virus levels didn't raise again, as normally happens after stopping antiretroviral therapy. At the time the case was reported, the São Paulo Patient had been completely virus-free for sixty-six weeks. Another four people who participated in the same clinical trial were not so lucky and relapsed, so the São Paulo Patient is only the third person ever to be cured of the infection. As yet, we have no answers to the questions of why this particular treatment worked for him, and whether the effects are going to be permanent.

A similar case was reported in 2014. The Mississippi Baby, a girl born of an infected mother, was treated immediately after birth with antiretrovirals. When the drugs were stopped eighteen months later, there was no sign of the virus. However, after twenty-seven months, the infection reappeared. This shows that the HIV can be hidden in the body for a long time without being detected and thus raises a note of caution for all the other patients currently considered to be 'cured'. Longer follow-ups will be needed before we can be certain of these apparent successes.

And the famous vaccine?

Despite all these treatments, a vaccine would be the most effective way to block the advance of the pandemic. But after more than three decades of research, we are still no closer to getting one, as the Nobel laureate and virologist David Baltimore pointed out a few years ago. Françoise Barré-Sinoussi has often declared that we are still a long way from having a vaccine, and that more basic laboratory work and clinical trials are needed if we are to have one sometime in the future. Some estimates venture that we won't have an effective vaccine for a decade; others are even more pessimistic. It's difficult to make predictions like this. We only need to recall the announcement of the US Health Secretary in 1984 telling us that the vaccine would be ready in two years.

The good news is that several vaccines are being clinically tested at present and are already in the advanced phases. Perhaps one of these will turn out to be effective sooner than expected. The big hurdle to be overcome, as I said at the beginning of this chapter, is the great variability of the virus and its ability to change fast enough to dodge the human body's immune responses. The perfect vaccine would need to yield antibodies that are different enough to be able to deal with all the forms that may keep appearing. Another factor is that HIV attacks precisely the best way we have of combating it: the immune system. However much we manage to activate it with a vaccine, if the virus has destroyed a considerable part of it, the body's response will never be sufficient.

The path to achieving a vaccine against HIV is strewn with failures. For example, Merck cancelled the clinical trials it was carrying out jointly with the National Institutes of Health of the United States because of the negative results they were getting in tests with one of the possible candidates, named Ad5. Research on this vaccine was abandoned in 2017. This was only the second vaccine that had come to be tested with humans in a study of this scale and, like its predecessor, it was a resounding failure. In 2020, the results for the candidate in the HVTN 702 trial were even more disappointing. But, a decade earlier, the RV 144 clinical trial had had limited success with a vaccine that showed some, but still insufficient, protection. More trials are continuing with modified versions of these vaccines, and results are expected in 2021.

This string of failures has been interpreted by some experts as a sign to go back to the laboratory and keep studying new possibilities and points of view that were different from the ones they'd been working with. The old lines of research, once apparently promising, hadn't lived up to expectations. Others, fearing even worse consequences, believe that all these setbacks are proof of the practical impossibility of ever finding a solution to the problem. The International AIDS Vaccine Initiative (IAVI), with headquarters in New York, coordinates the research efforts of laboratories that are working in the field around the world, as well as providing financial support. Some years ago, it was funding a good number of clinical trials, but now it's dividing the budget equally between testing and basic laboratory research. Nevertheless, at least forty more vaccines are in different phases of development, among them half a dozen in the advanced stages.

Given the considerable economic risk involved, most of the funding for research in the field comes from the public sector. In 2006, it was $883 million (with the United States contributing $225 million every year), while private contributions amounted to only $79 million. Investors don't like putting their money into a product that many see as not holding out any reasonable hope of success. Nevertheless, there are some private initiatives – such as the Ragon Institute in the Boston area, which is financed with $100 million donated by a former student of the Massachusetts Institute of Technology (MIT) who became a billionaire with a software company.

But there are still things left to try. Some people, after being infected, are able to produce antibodies against HIV that are powerful enough to prevent infection in laboratory animals. This small group of patients, who would have stronger defences, manages to block the virus without medical help. Some of them have been doing this for more than twenty-five years. It's believed that one in every 300 infected people is a so-called 'elite driver' who can beat the virus, and that about 5 per cent of HIV-positive patients never develop

Natural selection (with a bit of help from viruses)

The fact that certain primate species are often infected by the simian immunodeficiency virus (SIV) without ever developing any disease suggests that, at some point in history, SIV acted as a powerful selector.

Many years ago, there was most probably a population of 'elite drivers' among SIV-resistant monkeys, perhaps only 5 per cent of the total. Since the virus is very easily propagated, only the elite drivers would have survived. The rest would have died from the infection. Hence, present-day monkeys would be descendants of the original 5 per cent resistant ones.

This is an interesting way that species have of overcoming attacks by microbes, thanks to natural selection, and it's possible that it's happened several times throughout the ages, even among humans. Naturally, waiting for a few resistant individuals to survive and then to repopulate the planet isn't a viable solution in these times.

AIDS. It's possible that they hold the key to explaining how our immune system can fight AIDS. If we discover what makes them different from other people, the chances of finding a vaccine or some other way of dealing the virus would be very much better.

According to some studies, their blood has a large assortment of antibodies, more than 400 different types which, individually speaking, aren't very potent, but pulling together they are better at keeping HIV in check than the more specialized and aggressive antibodies. Most vaccines being studied at present are trying to induce these potent specific antibodies, which are of only four different types. Some experts now suggest that what's needed is to find a way to force the body to produce a greater variety of antibodies simultaneously, thus mimicking what seems to happen with the elite drivers. Other studies confirm that continually inducing low levels of antibodies might be more effective than trying to produce a powerful immune response.

In March 2020, an experimental vaccine generated these broadly neutralizing antibodies in human cells for the first time. This is only an early step in the process, a Phase I study, but it's a promising candidate that may perform better in further clinical trials.

Defence is the best attack

In the absence of a vaccine or cures, prevention is the best strategy right now, and this can only be achieved with broad involvement at the political and social levels. To prevent contagion by blood, several programmes are now under way to stop the reuse of syringes, and to test for the virus in blood donors. As for mother-to-child transmission, caesareans are performed to prevent contagion during birth, antiretrovirals

Radical prevention

In Indonesia, where AIDS is fast spreading, there was a proposal in 2008 to 'mark' HIV-positive people with a microchip so that they would always be monitored. At first, the aim was to apply the measure to 1–2 per cent of those infected and fine or even imprison them if it was found that they had purposely passed the virus on to someone else. The government shelved its plans when the international community harshly criticized it for not respecting human rights.

In 2009, an MP from Swaziland, where 26 per cent of the population is infected, suggested that HIV-positive people should be tattooed on the buttocks, a less technical version of the microchip, though equally discriminatory. The idea had been proposed earlier and, this time, it too was widely criticized.

are prescribed, and breastfeeding is avoided. These precautions have very good results.

The condom is still the most useful way of preventing sexual transmission. Despite strong campaigns over decades now, condom use isn't widespread enough in high-risk areas like sub-Saharan Africa or Southeast Asia. The morally grounded opposition of certain religious groups greatly compounds the problem.

Another area of prevention is that of *microbiocides*, in the form of creams applied to the vagina before intercourse. They have the advantage that the woman can use them without needing to ask for cooperation from her partner, an important fact in places where condom use isn't well accepted. Microbiocides form a barrier that physically prevents the virus from entering the cells of the vagina. These creams have become more important since it's been found that the walls of the vagina aren't such an effective barrier against entry of the virus as originally believed. The Bill & Melinda Gates Foundation donated $100 million so that this type of protection could be further studied and developed. The UK government contributed a further $30 million, but the pharmaceutical companies didn't invest much, so 90 per cent of the funding once again came from the public sector. However, numerous clinical trials are presently under way, and it is hoped that the number will double in the near future. The possibility of rectal microbiocides is also being studied. It's not yet known if they will end up being useful, as the walls of the rectum are more fragile than those of the vagina and are more difficult to protect.

The study of microbiocides had a setback in 2008 when the first large-scale trial for one called Carraguard turned out to be a less effective form of prevention than expected. Of the five clinical trials then under way, two had to be stopped, one of them because the cream was having the opposite effects to

Myth and reality: someone who is being treated for AIDS can't infect another person through sexual contact

This idea is encouraged by studies showing that antiretrovirals inhibit secretion of the virus in sexual fluids. In line with these findings, Switzerland announced that HIV-positive people didn't need to use condoms if they were being treated.

Published in summer 2008, another study using mathematical models showed that, although it's true that the risk of infection is lower, nobody should be advised to stop using protection because in a large enough population this would result in as many as four times more infections than there are at present.

those desired. One problem is that, owing to their contents, the creams can cause irritation and inflammation in the zones where they are applied, which can make it easier for HIV to enter. The first clinical trial with positive results was finally announced in February 2009. The so-called PRO2000 cut the risk of infection by 30 per cent. The data are still new and not very relevant in statistical terms, but they've given new hope to researchers.

One strategy that's clearly effective in obstructing the virus is circumcision. A study of 2007 demonstrated that circumcised men are 60 per cent less likely to be infected by AIDS. In other words, if the whole at-risk male population was circumcised, 60 per cent of deaths could be avoided in the next twenty years. The explanation is that the foreskin area is especially sensitive to the virus and many infections start right there. Yet, it seems that this benefit would only apply to heterosexuals, since studies show that it makes no significant difference among homosexuals. Neither does it seem that it protects the women with whom circumcised men have intercourse. One danger is that circumcision could give a false sense of security, which could lead to a diminished use of condoms. So, in the long run, it could be counterproductive.

An economical prevention?

In 2008, the World Bank came up with a new preventive strategy: paying people to protect themselves. The idea is simple. In order to get populations at risk to take precautions, they would be paid a sum of money every time they test negative for HIV. This would be supported with education and help in making the risks of infection known. A three-year clinical trial was carried out in Tanzania to see if the strategy, already the cause of considerable controversy, might really be useful.

Although it's a common intervention without too many complications, some African cultures oppose circumcision, which has hindered its introduction in places where it could be most effective. In countries like Niger, where the community is eminently Muslim (so men are circumcised and have less sexual freedom) the percentage of infected people is 0.7 per cent, while in Botswana, where circumcision levels are low and multiple sexual relations are commonplace, HIV-positive people represent 25 per cent of the population.

Where does the money come from?

The global expenditure on AIDS was $562.6 billion between 2000 and 2015. Investment in response to the issues caused by HIV in the US alone is now more than $28 billion per year. The President's Emergency Plan for AIDS Relief (PEPFAR), the programme responsible for distributing these funds, has managed to treat more than 2 million infected people worldwide. It's hoped that the number will soon be increased to 2.5 million, which would mean prevention of at least 12 million new infections. Between 2004 and 2007, PEPFAR managed to reduce the toll of AIDS deaths by 10 per cent in twelve African countries, at a cost of $2,700 for each life saved.

In the United States in 2007, presidential candidate Barack Obama announced during his electoral campaign that he would earmark a $1,000 million per year for PEPFAR but, when the crunch came in the form of the economic crisis, the sum had to be slashed. The same thing happened in other countries. Although the money invested in developing countries increased fivefold from 2002 to 2008, it was difficult thereafter to continue funding at the same rate. For example, in 2009, outlay for vaccine research dropped for the first time since 2000.

A gift with strings attached

PEPFAR's work began amidst controversy.

The rules for distributing the fund's money specified that a large part had to be allocated to promoting abstinence, and that recipients had to condemn prostitution. In practice, this meant that prostitutes couldn't be treated, even though they constituted one of the main at-risk populations.

It's been proved that such initiatives are of no use in stopping the pandemic. The US Congress eliminated this stipulation in 2008, but the programme continued to fund certain religious organizations that preached abstinence.

And here's an interesting fact: the first head of PEPFAR had to resign after it was discovered that he was linked to a prostitution ring.

In June 2009, PEPFAR had a new director and was faced with cuts in most of its programmes as a way of adapting to the new budget. The aim now was to allocate more resources to prevention than to treatment, contrary to what it had previously been doing. Moreover, part of the budget was to be devoted to combating malaria and tuberculosis, while also investing more in improving health and education in general.

Denialists: as dangerous as the virus

From the earliest days of the epidemic, there have been groups of people, eminent scientists among them, who refuse to believe that HIV causes AIDS. As early as 1984,

**Myth and reality:
vitamins are effective in combating AIDS.**

Although it's been pushed by some people who aren't fans of antiretrovirals, a vitamin treatment is neither a cure for AIDS nor a way of controlling it.

In June 2008, a South African judge ruled against promoting the use of vitamins as a substitute for antiretrovirals and a strategy for preventing and treating AIDS. This was another blow for those who, taking advantage of the fact that Thabo Mbeki was in power, were capitalizing on ignorance. Among them were two doctors, Matthias Rack and David Rasnick, who had been quick to set up a profitable snake oil business, selling vitamin complexes, claiming that they were effective and that antiretrovirals were toxic.

But, yes, it's true that malnutrition can favour development of the disease. Along the lines of this theory, a study of more than 1,000 pregnant women in Tanzania showed that a multivitamin treatment could slow the progress of the disease by up to 50 per cent in some cases. This could be especially advantageous in Africa, as vitamin treatments are cheap and could partially compensate for some of the deficiencies of antiretroviral treatments.

an article was published in a serious scientific journal claiming that AIDS was really an epidemic of collective hysteria. Logically speaking, denialism might have made sense when most of the details about the disease were still unknown but, with time and better information, the numbers of unbelievers have grown rather than diminished.

The denialists' theories have been demolished one by one, and time and time again (for example, it's still possible to see the rebuttals on the website www.aidstruth.org, which was active until 2015), so there's no longer any scientific basis to support the notion that HIV doesn't cause AIDS. Many denialists have ended up accepting reality and abandoning their ideas, but others obstinately keep ignoring the facts. The strategies of denialists have been compared with those of people who challenge the theory of evolution, others who claim that global warming isn't happening and still others who still believe that vaccines cause autism. Their common error is to cling only to the evidence that interests them and to ignore the many proofs that demonstrate the contrary.

Denialism could have been a mere anecdote if it weren't for the fact that it has been responsible for a great number of deaths in South Africa at the beginning of the twenty-first century. When Thabo Mbeki became president, he was faced with the fact that a very significant proportion of the population was HIV-positive. Aware of the problem that AIDS posed, he brought together a group of experts to advise him on the matter. But most of them were 'dissidents' and opposed to antiretrovirals, which happened to coincide with Mbeki's own views, so nobody listened to the few objective scientists in the advisory group. To make matters worse, Manto Tshabalala-Msimang, another zealous believer in the theory that HIV doesn't cause AIDS, was named minister of health. These political decisions led the South African government to promote quack remedies like consuming garlic and lemon juice, while opposing the distribution of antiretrovirals. The result was hundreds of thousands of avoidable deaths while Mbeki was in power: some 330,000 between 2000 and 2005, and that's not counting the 35,000 newborn babies with AIDS.

When Kgalema Motlanthe was elected president of South Africa in September 2008, after the resignation of Thabo Mbeki, Barbara Hogan replaced Tshabalala-Msimang as health minister. In one of her first declarations, Hogan said

They are everywhere

The denialists aren't only in Africa. There's a prominent group of them in the United States, including the Nobel laureate Kary Mullis (1944–2019), who was also well known for other controversial stands.

One influential denialist activist in the United States was Christine Maggiore, who, although HIV-positive when she became pregnant, and despite all the tests proving that drugs significantly hinder mother-to-child transmission, decided to refuse treatment because she didn't believe that HIV causes AIDS. She also decided to breastfeed, which is not recommended for HIV-positive mothers. Predictably, her daughter died of AIDS at the age of 3, and Maggiore herself died of it in 2008.

Maggiore campaigned and appeared in numerous magazines expounding her views until the very end of her life. The worst of it was that she had the support of certain *Sunday Times* journalists, which led *Nature* to publish an editorial denouncing the lamentable global health situation that could lead to crusades like Maggiore's. Nobody knows how many people died as a result of her obduracy.

she was ashamed of the enormous dimensions of the problem of AIDS in the country and made it clear that the era of denialism was over. The change of policy was welcomed and seen as a hopeful sign around the world. Nevertheless, AIDS denialists are still alive and kicking in many countries and, as the South African example testifies, they can have a calamitous influence on policies if they reach positions of power, causing countless victims. It is important to ensure that the right information about AIDS is made available with clear explanations for everyone, and that myths and falsehoods are patiently debunked.

9

Tuberculosis

People tend to speak of tuberculosis as if the word were associated with the typical disease of nineteenth-century romantic novels, where languid, pasty-faced characters coughed and coughed and ended their days in a sanitorium. It's no coincidence that consumptives of the day included writers like Balzac, Bécquer, Keats, Stevenson, Maupassant and Chekhov. Some, among them Kafka, Orwell and the Brontë sisters, died of the disease, as did many other artists until the middle of the twentieth century. It is believed that one in every seven people had tuberculosis in the mid-nineteenth century (and one in four people in London died of it at the beginning of the 1800s). But tuberculosis (or TB, as it's been called since the early twentieth century) has been with humans since long before that. Signs of tubercular lesions have been found in human bones that are more than 9,000 years old, and other traces have been discovered in Egyptian mummies dating back more than 5,000 years. But TB didn't start to become widespread until the growth of cities in the Middle Ages.

Although tuberculosis peaked between the eighteenth and nineteenth centuries, the idea that it's a plague of the past is totally mistaken. It's still a major health problem and one of the main causes of death by infection in adults. Worldwide, some 8 million people have tuberculosis every year, and 2 million won't recover. Russia, China, India and South Africa are the countries with most cases and the highest mortality rates, but the risk has spread to every corner of the planet. The resurgence of the disease this century is closely linked with AIDS, and one of the dangers is how quickly resistances to the usual drugs are appearing.

Koch's bacillus: an armoured microbe

Tuberculosis is caused by a microbe known as Koch's bacillus, named in honour of its German discoverer, Robert Koch, one of the scientists who has contributed most to the study of infections. Indeed, it's said that the 'golden age' of microbiology began in 1877 when Koch isolated the bacterium causing anthrax, as well as identifying the cause of cholera and, in 1882, describing the tuberculosis bacillus, for which he received a Nobel Prize in Physiology and Medicine in 1905. His legacy doesn't end there. His students went on to discover the microbes responsible for the main infectious diseases, for example diphtheria, typhus, meningitis, gonorrhoea, leprosy, syphilis and tetanus. Moreover, techniques for studying microbes developed by Koch are still being used today (see box).

Even when he erred, Koch made great strides forward. In 1890, he used extracts from the bacilli he had discovered in an attempt to cure tuberculosis. He called them *tuberculin*.

Koch's postulates

Robert Koch made another important contribution in the field of microbiology: he set out the four prerequisites that must be met in order to be sure that a microorganism is responsible for a disease.

1 It has to be present in all the sick people but not in healthy ones.
2 It must be possible to isolate it from the patient and cultivate it in the laboratory.
3 The isolated microorganism must be able to make a healthy person ill.
4 It must also be possible to isolate the microorganism from this second individual and to cultivate it in the laboratory once more.

As a treatment, they failed. Not only did they have no positive effect but, in some cases, they brought on an allergic reaction at the point where they had been injected. Later, it was found that this only happened if the patient had had previous contact with the bacillus. In other words, the tuberculin injection 'detected' people who'd been infected. Some years later, the French physician Charles Mantoux, turning this peculiarity to good effect, designed a test for diagnosing the disease and, with some variants, the Mantoux or PPD test is still being used today.

Koch's bacillus, whose technical name is *Mycobacterium tuberculosis*, is a bacterium from the same family as that causing leprosy. One of its characteristics is that it's very resistant as it's protected by a fatty layer that acts as a kind of armour to withstand a great number of toxic substances. Moreover, *Mycobacterium* can survive outside the body for hours before infecting someone else. This, and the fact that it can travel in saliva droplets, makes it as contagious as influenza can be. There's no need for bites, cuts or blood or fluid exchanges: sharing a room with a person with tuberculosis in the active phases can be enough for contagion to occur. Transmission is easier in places like hospitals and prisons where infected and healthy people have to share the same small spaces, especially if the sanitary conditions are substandard.

Normally, tuberculosis infections present no symptoms at first because the bacillus is 'dormant'. Unlike AIDS, the disease isn't contagious in this latent phase. But though it's inactive, our defences rarely manage to eliminate it completely. The main problem is that it can become activated at any time and, if this phase isn't treated, it's fatal in 50 per cent of the cases. Chronic inflammation appears in the area where the *Mycobacterium* has lodged, causing lesions called *granulomas* that destroy the organs where they appear. Well accommodated in the granulomas, the bacilli can survive within them for a long time.

In most cases of tuberculosis, the lungs are affected but the infection can also be seen in places like the brain or bones. Pulmonary tuberculosis can cause chest pain and a persistent cough, often with blood, together with fever, weight loss, pallor and fatigue, the classical symptoms described in literature.

A problem that comes back

Approximately a quarter of the world's population (some 2,000 million people) are infected by *Myobacterium tuberculosis*, but the active phase is only present in a small percentage (about 10 million cases). How can we know who will be in that group? First, it is supposed that there must be a genetic predisposition that makes some people more susceptible to the bacillus, and it's true that certain variants of genes called TLR8 and IL12B make their bearers more prone to picking up the *Mycobacterium*. It is also known that men are infected more easily than women, but not why this is so. Mortality is close to 1.5 million people per year.

Second, is the state of our defences. Normally the bacillus becomes activated in people whose immune system isn't very strong, for example children and the elderly. Recently, a third susceptible group has appeared, namely people with AIDS. We've seen that the main problem of an HIV infection is progressive destruction of the immune system. In addition, the virus blocks the lungs' specific defences for fighting the bacillus, thereby creating an ideal situation for the dormant *Mycobacterium* to reactivate and develop into tuberculosis.

It's mainly due to AIDS that there has been a significant rise in the number of tuberculosis patients since the early 1980s, when there were hardly any in developed countries. And it's still an upwards trend. In 2007, twice as many patients were diagnosed as having both AIDS and tuberculosis as during the previous year. In 2009, there were 1.4 million cases worldwide. In 2013, of the 9 million new tuberculosis cases, 1.1 million were diagnosed in HIV-positive patients and almost a third of those with this double infection will die as a result. In fact, 25 per cent of tuberculosis mortality is related to AIDS. At the beginning of this century, South Africa opened the first research centre studying the interactions between tuberculosis and AIDS. Partly funded by the Howard Hughes Medical Institute, an American nonprofit medical research organization, its location has been chosen as an area that's especially vulnerable to these diseases.

The threat of resistant tuberculosis

Since the mid-twentieth century, there have been some highly effective treatments against tuberculosis. The isoniazid drugs, discovered in the 1950s, were the first that proved to be effective against the bacillus. At present, a combination of specific antibiotics like rifampicin and isoniazid is the 'first-line' treatment. One peculiarity is that, in order to be sure that all the bacilli have been eliminated, at least two different drugs must be given for a long period (between six and twelve months), unlike what happens with other diseases whose treatment is briefer.

If antibiotics are effective, why is tuberculosis so

Primitive treatments

For a long time, there was no effective treatment for tuberculosis, although many different strategies with scant scientific basis had been tried. After the second half of the nineteenth century, patients were sent to sanitoriums to breathe 'pure air' because tuberculosis was understood to be a disease related to the poor conditions of hygiene in cities (and, in fact, the lower classes who lived in very unsanitary conditions were the most affected). Sanitoriums disappeared after the 1950s, when antibiotics were first used.

Before that, many other remedies had been tried, for example the 'royal touch' in the Middle Ages, when it was believed that monarchs had the power to cure this disease (and others), by a mere laying on of hands. Sessions were therefore organized where villagers were touched by the king, and, it was claimed, many were miraculously cured. This practice continued until the eighteenth century.

problematic? The looming threat is that variants of the bacillus that don't respond to the traditional antibiotics could appear. As early as spring 2009, the WHO saw this as a 'time bomb or a powder keg … a potentially explosive situation', and recommended that it had to be dealt with before these variants end up supplanting the drug-sensitive forms. In 2004, it was estimated that at least 0.5 million people were infected with resistant bacilli, and fifty-five countries around the world have already reported cases.

There are two main types of resistant *Mycobacteria*, the *multidrug resistant* (MDR) and *extensively drug-resistant* (XDR) forms, named in accordance with their resistance to fewer or more drugs. The latter type was discovered in 2005 and, of the patients infected with it, only between 12 and 60 per cent are cured, even when they've been treated. However, 90 per cent of people infected with the MDR type survive because these bacteria are sensitive to some antibiotics that still work. In 2006, there were almost 0.5 million new MDR infections and, in some parts of Asia, up to 70 per cent of new cases of tuberculosis are caused by MDR. In 2016, around 240,000 people died from MDR, according to the WHO. And there's yet a third group, the *totally drug-resistant* (TDR) bacilli, which don't respond to any of the four drugs used against tuberculosis. It's believed that the first of this group appeared in 2003, although no one was talking about them until 2012. They are still very uncommon.

Fortunately, XDR cases are also rare, although they've been detected in the great majority of countries. Between 1993 and 2007, only eighty-three were documented for the whole of the United States, with eighteen in the first year and only two in the last, thus showing a downwards trend. At first, 60 per cent were HIV-positive but this proportion dropped to 16 per cent in 2007, which is possibly a reflection of improvements in treatment and control of seropositive people. The former Soviet Union is one of the hotspots of the bacteria and, in Ukraine in particular, the XDR type causes 15 per cent of tuberculosis infections. In 2016, the WHO registered only 8,000 cases of XDR worldwide.

Nowadays, the best way of confronting the spread of MDR and XDR bacilli is to detect resistance quickly and isolate the patients. In the developed countries, techniques exist that can diagnose infection by these bacteria in less than twenty-four hours, but the system is too expensive for most poor countries. Work is being done with effective systems of detection that would only cost a few dollars per test.

New treatments, old treatments

Treatments for MDR have to be even longer than usual, which means more complications and a big hike in healthcare

Is there some solution?

In early 2009, a group of researchers at the Albert Einstein College of Medicine in New York discovered that two classic antibiotics could be effective against XDR. They immediately started clinical studies with patients to demonstrate the real effectiveness of the treatment. The solution to the lack of new antibiotics for treating tuberculosis could lie in being imaginative and testing combinations of existing drugs of proven effectiveness against other microorganisms.

Another advance is the drug called TMC207 which, in the first clinical trials in June 2009, showed that it was quicker in eliminating resistant bacilli. TMC207 acts by means of a mechanism that differs from those in drugs used so far and could be an important treatment in future.

costs. The few antibiotics that still work with MDR are by no means new ones. Some, like capreomycin and cycloserine, were discovered in the 1950s. But because of their significant side effects (neurological damage and psychosis in 1 per cent of people who take cycloserine) or problems with administering them (capreomycin must be injected), no one was using them. And this is precisely why they are so effective. It's so long since they've been used that the bacteria haven't had a chance to develop resistance. In September 2008, it was found that a drug called R207910, which was still in the experimental phases of testing as a possible treatment for MDR, could eliminate 95 per cent of the dormant bacteria. Alternatively, new antibiotics are constantly being studied with the aim of eradicating XDR and TDR.

Activism and private nonprofit initiatives are also crucial in efforts to control tuberculosis. For example, with help from the Bill & Melinda Gates Foundation, China launched an initiative in April 2009 to fight tuberculosis across the country. The programme included testing new drugs against resistant bacteria and new ways of detecting them to enable faster and more effective treatment. China and the Foundation are also carrying out research into possible new drugs based on traditional remedies. Among the plants customarily used in Chinese medicine and now being studied, some twenty-four candidates with anti-tuberculosis effects have been identified.

Over the course of the twentieth century, tuberculosis became an easy disease to control because of antibiotics. With the appearance of MDR, XDR and TDR, the situation has completely changed. If the resistant bacilli start spreading, which is very possible with migratory movements from countries of the East to Western Europe, we could be faced with a highly contagious pandemic with no treatment available. The solution is closer control of patients, making sure that they receive the treatment they need as soon as possible, and that they continue with it for the whole time prescribed. But it is also necessary to keep researching to find new treatments and, in particular, a vaccine.

Another disease with no vaccine

Although Koch's bacillus isn't able to keep changing, unlike the AIDS and influenza viruses, no vaccine that is truly effective against tuberculosis has been discovered yet. The only one that exists, BCG (*Bacille Calmette-Guérin*) slows the progress of the disease to some extent, but doesn't prevent it (giving only 20 per cent protection at most). Its particularity is that it's not made with the human tuberculosis bacterium but from that of cows (*Mycobacterium bovis*). Although it is understood that the immunity it confers isn't complete – even if the two types of bacteria are very similar – BCG is widely used around the world, especially to protect children in zones where the risk is higher.

The tuberculosis vaccine is another field where governments have invested little and NGOs have had to intervene. In February 2004, the Bill & Melinda Gates Foundation donated almost $83 million to incentivize the search for a more effective vaccine. This is a considerable sum, especially as it represents twice what was being spent around the world in the field. The solution might be improvement of already-existing vaccines. In 2009, a group of scientists in Texas announced that they had obtained a more effective version of BCG. If it's administered together with a dose of rapamycin (an anti-inflammatory used as an anti-cancer agent, and to prevent rejection after transplants) it enables BCG to destroy ten times more bacilli.

The tuberculosis that comes from cows

If cows have their own *Mycobacterium*, can milk from an infected animal cause tuberculosis? It's true that, before the discovery of pasteurization, bovine tuberculosis could pass to humans through dairy products. But, nowadays, cows are rigorously monitored. A sick cow is immediately sacrificed to avoid contagion and, moreover, cows that are to be exported have to undergo tests to prove that they haven't been infected in the previous thirty days.

Cleaning up milk

Pasteurization is a system invented by Louis Pasteur in 1862 with the aim of reducing the number of microorganisms in food and, in particular, improving the shelf life of beer and wine. It's different from sterilization, which seeks to eliminate absolutely every trace of microorganisms. This can't be done with food because it would destroy proteins. Milk, for example, curdles or 'spoils' if it's boiled with a view to sterilizing it. Pasteurization, then, uses temperatures below boiling point. Present-day techniques can eliminate up to 99.999 per cent of the microorganisms, including *M. tuberculosis*.

The United Kingdom allocates about £100 million per annum for controlling bovine tuberculosis. Approximately thirty people are infected around the country every year. In some of these cases, those of elderly people, it's thought that this could be due to reactivation of the virus they've harboured for a long time, since the days of drinking unpasteurized milk.

Bovine tuberculosis represents economic losses for the

livestock sector, but the danger of the infection being passed on to humans is minimal, although there are occasional cases among farmers who have direct contact with cows. The experts say that if the infected animals are sacrificed quickly, there's no danger that the virus will gather enough 'strength' to make the leap to humans in any significant numbers.

10

Malaria

Between 350 and 500 million people are infected with malaria every year and 1 million of them, mostly children, will die. It's calculated that someone dies of malaria every thirty seconds, and that's not counting the cases where it has aggravated previous infections. At present, 60 per cent of cases are to be found in sub-Saharan Africa, a quarter of them in Congo and Nigeria.

Since more than a decade ago, when the Bill & Melinda Gates Foundation once again raised the question of eradication (a term that had been dropped some time earlier), there have been renewed efforts in combating malaria. An initial date set for declaring victory over the disease was 2025, though it seems that this probably won't happen. In any case, right now is a golden age for malaria research, and the weapons we have at present could be enough to eliminate it in the near future. We only need to find a way to apply them where they are needed most, but this is no easy task. Science has done some of the work, but the next step is to find a way of putting the advances to good use. Some important innovations are still lacking as is, once again, an effective vaccine.

All because of a mosquito

Malaria has been with us for millennia. Traces have been found in Egyptian mummies dating back to 3000 BCE, and it's mentioned in Chinese medicinal treatises of 2700 BCE. The main symptoms are fever, joint pains, vomiting, anaemia and even convulsions. It frequently presents with episodes lasting from between four to six hours, of suddenly feeling cold and stiff, followed by fever and profuse sweating. This can happen every two or three days. Severe cases usually appear one or two weeks after infection and can lead to coma or death, sometimes in just a few hours. The mortality rate is between 10 and 20 per cent, and children who survive can have sequelae affecting their development. Infection in the brain accounts for some of the child victims (and, indeed, cerebral malaria kills in 20 per cent of cases).

Malaria isn't caused by a bacterium, or by a virus either, but by a kind of microbe called protozoan, which is related to algae and amoebae. The protozoan responsible for malaria is of the genus *Plasmodium* and was discovered at the end of the nineteenth century. In 2002, the genome of one of the four malaria *Plasmodia* (known as *falciparum*) was sequenced, as was another (*vivax*) in 2008. Our ignorance about these microorganisms is clear when we face the fact that, even when we've been able to read their DNA, we still don't understand the function of many of their genes.

The microbe enters the body through a mosquito bite. Inside the mosquito and, specifically, tucked away in its saliva glands, the *Plasmodium* has an ideal haven to grow, develop and divide, but it also likes a change of residence. Once the

Mosquitoes are gourmets too

Not everyone has the same chances of being bitten by a mosquito. This may sound like an old wives' tale, but it's been scientifically demonstrated. Some people are definitely more likely to get malaria than others.

Who is most at risk? According to studies on the matter, mosquitoes prefer to bite pregnant women, people with a low body mass index (the slimmer ones), and ... people with smelly feet. These reasons for these odd preferences are still a mystery.

mosquito bite lets it get into a human, it goes straight to the liver, where it multiplies before moving into the bloodstream. The cycle is closed if another mosquito bites the infected person and thereby captures the *Plasmodia* circulating in the blood. It then transmits the parasite to a different person, with another bite, and so on. The infection can be latent and not appear until months or even years after the first mosquito bite.

Mosquitoes that transmit malaria are of the genus *Anopheles*, of which there are fifty different species. Many of them aren't harmful, and a lot of mosquitoes within one and

To catch a mosquito

In order to collect data on populations of *Anopheles* mosquitoes in a certain zone, and its bite frequency, the usual technique used by researchers is the 'human landing capture'. A volunteer sits quietly, trousers raised to the knees, waiting patiently for a mosquito to bite, whereupon a colleague captures it using a device with a rubber suction tube. It may sound basic, but it's a very effective method.

the same species won't actually transmit the disease. Hence, there must be a genetic determinant which means that some mosquitoes can infect people and others can't. If we could discover what it is, we would be well on the way to controlling the spread of the disease.

Thanks to a series of genetic studies, it has been possible to deduce that malaria originated in monkeys, as did AIDS. It was transmitted to humans at least 10,000 years ago, possibly because of one mosquito bite. It spread through tropical zones and then around the world about 5,000 years ago, coinciding with the beginnings of agriculture.

Goodwill is not enough

Efforts to curb malaria have had very little success so far. In 1955, the WHO initiated the first global campaign, which fizzled out in the 1960s. Then, Roll Back Malaria, a group

---

Myth and reality

An oft-repeated myth is that money given to treat diseases in developing countries disappears before reaching those who need it. In the vast majority of cases, this isn't so.

One exception is Uganda. A report from 2006 demonstrated that $45.3 million assigned to the country by the Global Fund to Fight AIDS, Tuberculosis and Malaria had gone missing thanks to corruption. The money had ended up in the pockets of officials and middle-management people through false NGOs and invoices for nonexistent services.

Uganda doesn't have either the money or the resources to prosecute all the fraudsters, so only a small proportion of the stolen funds was recovered.

consisting of governments, NGOs and some individuals, began its campaign in 1998 with the promise of cutting the number of malaria cases by half before 2010, but progress was slower than expected. The 2000 Abuja Declaration on Roll Back Malaria in Africa, signed by the heads of state of several African countries, didn't achieve much either. The aim of the UN's Millennium Development Goals was more modest and attainable: to stop growth in the number of cases of malaria by 2015. This goal was partly achieved.

The human and economic resources invested in recent years seem to suggest that, nowadays, there's considerable interest in beating malaria. In 2007 alone, $1,500 million were allocated for the cause. In September 2008, Roll Back Malaria announced a Global Malaria Action Plan, estimating

A medicinal cocktail

Gin and tonic started out as having a purely medicinal function. Tonic was made of carbonated water infused with a therapeutic dose of quinine, which was the first known treatment against malaria. Its function was preventive. The problem was its strong, bitter taste, which so repulsed British soldiers stationed in India in the nineteenth century that they refused to take the medicine, so the health problems persisted. But someone found the solution: if gin was added to the tonic, much of the bitter taste was neutralized. Thereafter, the quinine treatment, in the form of gin and tonic, became very popular among the soldiers.

The brands of tonic being marketed today contain much less quinine (between 0.25 per cent and 0.50 per cent of the original amount) and a lot more sugar (or artificial sweetener), so they offer no protection against malaria. But, yes, they are still good for making gin and tonic.

that more than $6,000 million were needed to get it under way. It was launched in the UN General Assembly head-quarters with the participation of Bono, lead singer of the rock band U2. Half the money needed was immediately raised with help from the Bill & Melinda Gates Foundation (presently the biggest private donor in research into malaria), the World Bank and the Global Fund to Fight AIDS, Tuberculosis and Malaria. The ambitious goal of the Action Plan is, first, to reduce the death toll to practically zero and then, little by little, to eradicate malaria from all the countries where it's endemic. Many experts say that this won't be possible in the next fifty years, even if efforts and donations continue to increase.

The treatment and how to get it to people who need it

By 1999, malaria treatment programmes in Africa were failing, and a large number of plasmodia had become resistant to the usual drugs (chloroquine and sulfadoxine/pyrimethamine). However, the situation has now improved. Artemisinin, obtained in 1972 by Dr Tu Youyou working with a traditional Chinese remedy (which earned her a Nobel Prize in Physiology or Medicine in 2015), is a very effective treatment with few side effects. Artemisinin-based combination therapies (ACT), which include other antimalarials in the mix, are presently being given over three days, and this eliminates the disease in 95 per cent of cases.

Although there's an effective cure, people keep dying of malaria for the same reason as they die of tuberculosis: access to drugs is a long way from being universal. According to WHO data from 2006, only 23 per cent of children in Africa sleep under a mosquito net – a strategy that, as we shall see, is very effective as prevention – and only 3 per cent of the population has access to ACTs.

To begin with, ACTs are sixty times more expensive than other older, less effective treatments. To take Uganda as an example, fewer than 14 per cent of private outlets have ACTs. Instead, they offer outdated and almost useless drugs like chloroquine, and even fake medicines, but at very accessible prices. To this, it must be added that the information supplied to consumers is almost nonexistent, which often means that people buy cheaper pills without suspecting that they will have no effect. Unless a way is found for distributors to buy ACTs more cheaply from the manufacturers, the problem will persist.

A new distribution system is therefore being studied. Instead of giving governments funds so they can buy medicines from the companies and then supply them to their clinics, the donors will hand the money directly to the pharmaceutical companies, with the idea that they will sell the drugs at lower prices. Hence, the really effective products would be as cheap or cheaper than the others, and sick people could buy them more easily from small pharmacies. This financing mechanism, called Affordable Medicines Facility-malaria (AMFm), started out with $225 million donated by the UK government and a private foundation.

Has the time of resistances come?

As early as 2006, the WHO recommended that the pharmaceutical companies should stop selling artemisinin as a single drug (called *monotherapy*) and to change definitively to ACTs, which is a much more effective way of avoiding resistances. Many of the manufacturers didn't respect this guideline because monotherapies are cheaper to make and easier to sell. This poses a significant danger because, if plasmodia that are insensitive to artemisinin start appearing, there's no other equally good alternative for defeating them right now. When the situation hadn't changed by 2009, the WHO took sterner action and issued a communique demanding that governments should ban the companies from marketing artemisinin as a monotherapy.

Not long before this, the first resistances had been seen in Cambodia. In December 2008, there were reports of a zone with cases in which malaria wasn't disappearing with any treatment. The following May, the news broke that two clinical trials had demonstrated the existence of a type of malaria

Phases of a clinical study

0   First tests in humans. A single dose of the drug is given in a concentration below what is thought will really be effective. 10–15 healthy volunteers.

I   Different concentrations of the drug are given in a hospital setting for a prolonged period, to evaluate side effects. 20–80 volunteers, normally healthy.

II Once it is established that the drug is safe, its positive effects are evaluated, while Phase I studies continue in larger groups. 20–300 volunteers, both healthy and sick.

III Effectiveness is compared with that of other already approved treatments. Simultaneous studies in more than one centre, often in different countries. A drug that satisfactorily passes a couple of Phase III studies is often approved for public use. 300–3,000 volunteers.

IV Long-term studies once the drug is marketed keep checking on its safety and effectiveness. Some drugs have been withdrawn from the market when a Phase IV study detects unanticipated problems that weren't picked up earlier.

that didn't respond to artemisinin. The scientific articles that should have described these studies in more detail weren't made public and the WHO website deleted all references to them, immediately casting doubt on the veracity of the story. But on 29 July 2009, the information was officially confirmed, and details were made available to the public. The resistance wasn't total, but artemisinin took longer than usual to eliminate the microbes. It was feared that resistance would appear in Africa where malaria is very common, and more people could be affected.

Some scientists have been warning of these possible resistances for a long time but, owing to difficulties in interpreting the data, they've often been ignored. One pertinent factor is that it was in this same region of Asia that resistance to chloroquine first appeared long ago.

The controversial SPf66 vaccine

What's the current state of the antimalarial vaccine? Produced by the Colombian researcher Manuel Elkin Patarroyo in 1987, the first to be tested in a population was called SPf66. He ceded the rights of the vaccine to the WHO in 1993 after refusing offers from several pharmaceutical companies. Since then, he's received many international awards in recognition of this gesture.

In the Phase I studies, the vaccine showed an efficiency of 75 per cent, but when the trials moved on to Phase II and Phase III at the end of the 1990s, the results fell to 30 per cent and 60 per cent respectively. Some studies even claimed it had no effect. The results, therefore, were contradictory and not at all hopeful. Many subsequent studies were carried out with large numbers of people, but there's still no convincing evidence to show that the vaccine is effective, so most experts have stopped believing in it and prefer to focus their efforts on a new generation.

In fact, Patarroyo's studies were controversial from the start, as he was accused of testing the vaccine with too many volunteers without having completed the necessary preliminary studies to ascertain its effectiveness and safety.

Myth and reality

Did Patarroyo's vaccine fail because of a plot hatched by the pharmaceutical companies that didn't want an independent researcher to get the benefits?

This is one of the myths that is most frequently raised when people talk about SPf66. The truth is simple. The vaccine didn't manage to pass the necessary tests in order to be declared successful, and now it seems that there are better options.

Dr Pedro Alonso, director of the WHO's Global Malaria Programme commented that it's absurd to believe in a boycott by companies that want to wipe a competitor off the map. The problem is just the opposite: since they don't see a product like this as being very profitable, they have no interest in investing in the field. GSK, for example isn't expecting big profits from its RTS,S vaccine and has announced that its aim is to try to make it accessible to the people who need it most.

The army is also researching

Work on the malaria vaccine was initially greatly boosted by research carried out by the US Army. Since the Vietnam War, the government has invested large sums of money in trying to find ways of protecting its soldiers from malaria when they are stationed in tropical countries. Over the years, several vaccines have been studied, among them NYVAC-Pf7 and [NANP]19-5.1, and work is presently being done on as many as thirty different types.

GSK has a vaccine called RTS,S, which started a Phase III study (between 12,000 and 16,000 children in Africa) in September 2008, and this is the one that's gone farthest to date. Once again, the Bill & Melinda Gates Foundation has helped with funding, and GSK has contributed $500 million since research began.

The first laboratory experiments leading to the production of RTS,S began in the 1970s. Military studies in 1987 demonstrated that an early form of this vaccine provided a certain degree of immunity. Of the six researchers who volunteered to test it on themselves by getting bitten by a swarm of infected mosquitoes, five got malaria and one was spared. Teams in the army laboratories, led by Dr Rip Ballou and working with GSK teams headed by Dr Joe Cohen, managed to improve the vaccine to the point it has reached in its current form. Whether RTS,S prevents infections or merely delays them for some years, or even how long the supposed protection lasts, are still unanswered questions, but the results are encouraging.

However, the protection provided by RTS,S is partial (working in only 50 per cent of cases) and, moreover, four injections are needed to achieve immunity. Nevertheless, it was approved in 2015 and is marketed with the name of Mosquirix, although it isn't recommended for small children, who constitute one of the groups most affected by the disease. While it is starting to be used in some African countries, another generation of vaccines is also being studied. But, at present there's no other candidate in the advanced stages of testing that has proved to be better than RTS,S.

Against the insects:
mosquito nets and genetic engineering

Apart from treatment and vaccines, the simplest prevention methods can have a big impact in malaria control, as we've seen with other major infectious diseases. Gambia is one example. An initiative that began in 2003 has brought about a 90 per cent reduction in the country's malaria deaths, mainly because of insecticides, mosquito nets and preventive treatments for children. And 50 per cent of those under the age of 5 now sleep protected by a mosquito net.

Some years ago, the Zambian government launched an ambitious plan to cut the cases of malaria by 75 per cent, and deaths have already dropped by 30 per cent. Once again, using mosquito nets and insecticides, as well as giving preventive treatment to pregnant women and ACT treatment within twenty-four hours of infection, are having a significant effect. In the last few years, the impact of malaria has declined considerably in other African countries like Eritrea and Rwanda, and the island of Zanzibar. The improvements range between 50 and 75 per cent simply because people are using mosquito nets and there's better access to drugs. The figures show that, since 2000, mosquito nets alone have cut infection rates by half in the countries where they are being used.

Since new techniques designed to attack the vector insects have turned out to be a highly effective form of prevention, they are also being studied. For example, if a mosquito unable to transmit *Plasmodia* could compete with undoctored *Anopheles* mosquitoes, the population capable of infecting humans would end up diminishing or disappearing. With the new tools of genetic engineering, it's possible to 'manufacture' these resistant mosquitoes in a laboratory. Early experiments have also been carried out with mosquitoes infected by a bacterium that makes them sterile, which means that the overall population would decline when they are released into a controlled zone. Laboratory mosquitoes most probably won't be the solution to malaria but, combined with other improvements in treatments and prevention, they could be another important weapon in the struggle.

Another option is to act against the bacteria that normally infect the *Anopheles* mosquito. As with humans, the *Anopheles* mosquito has a flora of bacteria living in harmony with it. In the case of malaria, these 'good' bacteria would help to prevent the mosquito from being infected by plasmodia. Some scientists are looking into the possibility of increasing the concentration of these bacteria in the insect's intestines to improve its defences.

Global action

The paradox of malaria is that, although we don't yet have a vaccine, the treatment is effective and simple prevention measures also have good results. On paper, there should be no more victims. But, as I said, these benefits haven't been put into practice, mostly because of the difficulty of ensuring that everyone has access to the advances being made in the field. Science alone isn't enough to defeat infectious diseases. Well-planned social intervention is also needed. And this is why some experts keep saying that, besides investing money in the laboratory and encouraging research into new drugs and vaccines, we must make the most of all the tools we already have.

Dr Jordi Gómez i Prat, head of the Unit of Tropical Medicine and International Health, in Drassanes, Barcelona, is engaged in the struggle against malaria in Jaú National

Park in the heart of the Amazon rainforest in Brazil. His experience has demonstrated that the battle against malaria must be specifically adapted to each affected zone. First and foremost, it is necessary to be well informed about the place concerned so as to understand what strategies might be most useful, and to know how to locate the places where, and the times when, the disease is most frequently transmitted. This could lead to a change of habits, which can have a big impact on health. For example, if it is found that most infections can be traced to the river at certain hours, then other fishing places and other times of day are considered. At the same time, it's necessary to work towards improvement in general health, and to struggle against malnutrition and other diseases that can gravely complicate the effects of malaria.

Working directly with the affected community is also essential. This means informing the people about preventive measures and involving them in the project, so they can know how to detect the disease, understand that it really is a matter of life and death, and act against it more quickly. With measures like these, which don't cost large amounts of money, many of the serious cases can be avoided. Dr Gómez i Prat's team, for example, has published educational books addressed to local populations, explaining in clear, understandable terms, complete with drawings and testimonies from children, how to fight malaria.

One of the crucial factors is fast diagnosis. The longer it takes to identify the disease, the more likely contagion of other people will be, in addition to putting the sick person at risk. People must therefore be trained to use a microscope to identify the plasmodium, and well-equipped health centres should be set up in the most vulnerable areas. The aim is that everyone who presents with fever would have a diagnosis in less than twenty-four hours. But Jordi Gómez i Prat is well aware that there is still a long way to go before everyone can have a diagnosis and treatment. In the Jaú area there are two doctors for an area almost as big as the United Kingdom, without roads, so they often have to travel by canoe, which means that it's very important to train local inhabitants so they can become involved in detecting and treating the disease. Intelligent use of available resources, guided by someone who knowns the specific problems of each region, can have significant results. 'Neurons are more necessary than money', Gómez i Prat says, 'and we must manage to get governments involved.'[15]

A tropical disease only?

Malaria is mostly seen in developing countries, humid climates and areas where poverty is rife. But not long ago, it was much more widespread. It wasn't until the mid-twentieth century that it was eradicated in Europe and North America. It was the Italians who gave the disease its present name, from *mal aria* (bad air), as they believed it was transmitted by miasmas coming off swamps. In 1940, Spain registered 5,000 victims. Malaria has disappeared in these climes mostly because the mosquitoes' breeding grounds (marshy areas, stagnant water, and so on) were eliminated.

So, if Southern Europe provides the right conditions for the *Anopheles* mosquito to thrive, it's not found exclusively in tropical areas. Is there any danger, then, that malaria could come back to this part of the world in the form of an epidemic? In principle, it can extend to developed countries because of frequent travel to zones where it's endemic, but

15 From an interview by the author with Jordi Gómez i Prat [translation: JW].

we should recall that the disease isn't transmitted between humans. The mosquito has to be the vector. Tourism is, in fact, responsible for the sporadic cases we see in Europe, especially because proper precautions are frequently not taken. It's calculated that, in 2004, more than 2.4 million people from the United Kingdom visited places where malaria is endemic, many of them migrants visiting their families. Only 42 per cent of these people had preventive treatment. Between 1989 and 2005, of the cases of malaria recorded in Barcelona, 96 per cent hadn't completed the preventive treatment. There were almost 1,600 cases of infection and six people, all of them tourists, died. In other words, the mortality rate is nearly 4 per cent. Lack of awareness and ignorance among Europeans about the symptoms of malaria means that many patients don't get to start the treatment until the disease is already in the advanced stages.

Bill Gates's unfunny joke

In February 2009, Bill Gates was giving a lecture in California at an event organized by his foundation. In order to illustrate how terrible the impact of malaria is, he released some mosquitoes (seven, it seems) onto the audience, telling them that, 'there's no reason only poor people should have the experience' of fear of infection.

Only then did he assure them that the mosquitoes weren't plasmodium bearers. Nevertheless, the audience got quite a scare.

It often happens that travel agencies, loath to recommend vaccines and preventive treatments because they think it could affect tourism, don't give the necessary warnings. Jordi Gómez i Prat recommends that people who want to travel to any countries where malaria is endemic should always consult an expert in tropical diseases. 'If you know the risks, you can act accordingly and protect yourself better.' If you are informed about how malaria is transmitted, planning preventive measures is easier, and the risks are then almost zero. 'It's like looking both ways before you cross the road', he says.[16]

Tourists are not the only problem; another is 'airport malaria', which appears when a mosquito stows away on a plane leaving a zone where malaria is endemic and going to a country that's free of it (normally Europe or North America). It's known that *Anopheles* mosquitoes catch planes because, in a radius of a couple of kilometres around international airports (for example, in New York and Los Angeles), there are often individual cases of malaria, especially in warm weather when the mosquitoes have better chances of thriving. So, we shouldn't be surprised to learn that cases of malaria have recently been seen even in places like Switzerland. The fact that the whole planet is affected by global warming only increases the chances that the mosquito will spread, and this doesn't only apply to malaria but also to other insect-borne diseases, for example dengue fever. In theory, this could cause future epidemics of tropical diseases outside the endemic zones.

16 See footnote 15 on p. 270.

Epilogue

When I presented the first draft of this project to my Catalan publishers a few years ago, they were surprised to find that, in the summary of one of the chapters, I confidently stated that we would see a new pandemic before long. I also told them about epidemics that kill millions of people, increasingly aggressive viruses, bacteria that are no longer responding to treatments, terrifying weapons that are within the reach of almost anybody, and new diseases appearing out of the blue against which we've got no way of defending ourselves. They thought that maybe I was a little alarmist. But this is the reality and, unfortunately, the appearance of COVID-19 has confirmed my predictions. The fact that the general public isn't fully aware of the role infections have played in the history of humanity, and will keep playing in its future, is one of the reasons that prompted me to write this book.

What I've described in these pages is happening all around us and we can't ignore it. These aren't just theories and predictions about a future we will never see. I myself have witnessed how a whole New York hospital building was shut down for hours in 2001 because of panic over a biological weapons attack after someone dropped a sugary doughnut in the lobby leaving behind a white powder that was mistaken for anthrax spores. Next time it could really be anthrax.

I had the idea of writing about these matters long before the appearance of the COVID-19 pandemic showed us that we aren't immune to pandemics in the twenty-first century. After my previous attempts at popular science writing, I started wondering about which scientific field might interest readers. Not only that, I wanted to find areas which, because of their importance for our health, frequently had media coverage but also raised enough doubts and questions among the public to justify a scientist's attempts to offer comprehensible explanations. That wasn't too difficult.

During my time in New York, researching into cancer and cellular ageing, I also had the opportunity to work with a group of scientists of international renown in the field of infectious diseases, some of whom appear in this book. At the time, it was a totally new field for me, but their enthusiasm was contagious, and I threw myself into learning everything I could about microbes. Several jointly authored articles published in specialist journals eventually resulted from that desire to discover new things, as well as a fascination for the subject that has lasted to the present day. I hope to have infected my readers a little with the allure of crossing boundaries, and also to have made the mysterious world of microorganisms a bit better known.

We can only marvel at the biological perfection of the simplest life forms that exist. We often ignore them, or despise them, but their ability to survive against all odds is something humans will always envy. And this is why they've held sway over us for millennia. In the last century and a half, we've been able to wrest some control over the situation, but we are still subject to their tyranny and it is important never to forget that. New diseases with the potential to wipe us off the face of the Earth are constantly appearing. We learn how to curb some of them, but others take us by surprise and disappear before we can marshal our defences. If a virus transmitted as fast as flu or COVID-19 and with something approaching the mortality of Ebola were one day to appear – and this possibility isn't as remote as we would like to imagine – we will have to fight with all our might to survive as a species. We would do well to be prepared.

There is one thing we should be very clear about: we are all in the same boat. We can't ignore an epidemic just because it's happening thousands of kilometres away from where we live. We need to know how to detect outbreaks of serious diseases quickly so we can stop them and eradicate them before they spread all around the planet. We can't keep designing strategies at the state level alone, but must do so everywhere in the world and in unison. This means investing resources, especially in developing countries.

The COVID-19 pandemic has been a test for our global defence systems. We've seen that there's a lot of room for improvement but also that we are starting to coordinate and act more efficiently now. Next time – and there will certainly be a next time – it's to be hoped that we will do better. Information is now travelling faster than ever, and we only need to make governments throughout the world understand that, if we all act together, we have the chance of saving millions of lives. Fortunately, this necessary vision of humans uniting against a common enemy is becoming more and more generalized.

The twenty-first century could also be the time of our ceasing to witness how millions of people die of diseases against which we've had effective measures for some time. It seems that this fact has now registered in the right places, and programmes designed to help Africa, the Americas and Asia escape from the grip of microbes are beginning to take effect. It's to be hoped that medicines and vaccines will soon reach everyone who needs them, no matter where they are.

As I said at the outset, we share Earth with microorganisms. In fact, it's their planet. We are just distant relatives who have been invited to the party. If we want to keep living here, we have to learn to set limits. We have the tools and intelligence to do this. So, now let's see if we can.

Glossary

Antibiotic: a substance that kills a bacterium or hinders its growth. Many are obtained from microorganisms, while others are laboratory modifications of natural products.

Antibodies: proteins that recognize specific parts of the organisms that infect us and activate other defence mechanisms. Antibodies are part of our immune system. Vaccines act by inducing the production of specific antibodies against a microbe so the body will be better prepared if there is an infection.

Antigens: specific structures of a microorganism that are recognized by antibodies. Antigens, isolated and purified, are used as vaccines because they activate the immune system.

Antiretrovirals: antivirals specifically used against HIV. They are the treatment of choice for preventing the appearance of AIDS in people infected by the virus.

Antivirals: drugs that stop growth of a virus. They are of limited effectiveness and are therefore less able to cure viral infections.

Attenuated: used of a living microorganism that has been modified to stop it from causing any disease. Attenuated microbes are used for certain types of vaccines.

Bacilli: rod-shaped bacteria.

Binary fission: the process by which a bacterium divides into two exactly equal parts.

Buboes: swollen inflamed lymph nodes resulting from infection by *Yersinia pestis* and leading to the typical tumours of bubonic plague.

Carriers: infected individuals who don't develop the disease though they can infect other people.

CDC: Centers for Disease Control and Prevention of the US government, responsible for coordinating responses to outbreaks of infectious diseases, *inter alia*.

Cocci: bacteria that are rounded in form.

Cytokines: chemical substances released by the human body to 'wake up' its defences when faced by an invader. If too many are produced, an excessive inflammatory reaction occurs with an accumulation of fluids in the wrong places, which can prevent the organs from functioning and, in extreme cases, cause death.

Endemic: describes the situation when an infectious disease is constantly present in a region without an overall increase or decrease in the number of cases.

Epidemic: a higher number than usual of infected people. The word usually describes an outbreak that has spread to affect quite a large population.

Granuloma: a lesion formed by an accumulation of immune cells that try to isolate an alien substance they haven't been able to eliminate. Tuberculosis and leprosy are two infections that cause granulomas.

HAART: Highly Active Antiretroviral Therapy, a combination of at least three antiretrovirals, and of at least two different types, the currently used treatment for AIDS.

Haemagglutinin: a protein of the capsule of a virus enabling it to attach itself to the cells of the organism it infects. There are sixteen types and it's one of the antigens used to produce vaccines. Abbreviated as H.

Immune system: a defence network formed by tissues, cells, proteins and other substances that work in a well-coordinated fashion to stop anything they detect as alien. The *innate immune system* attacks invaders nonspecifically, and the *adaptive immune system* is geared to attack each specific invader.

Immunization: activation of a person's immune system; for example, by means of a vaccine, to make it impervious to a microbe.

Inactivity: the state of a microorganism that's been killed to be used for a vaccine.

Leucocytes (or white blood cells): the blood cells tasked with fighting infections.

Lipodystrophy: a disorder affecting the distribution of body fats. It's common among HIV-positive people who are being treated with antiretrovirals. They lose fat on the face and in extremities and accumulate it on the torso, to the point of considerable deformity.

Lymphocytes: a type of leucocyte that, among other things, produces antibodies.

MDR (multidrug resistant): designating bacteria that are resistant to more than one antibiotic.

Microbe: a microorganism.

Microbiocides: creams that are applied the vagina before sexual intercourse with the aim of preventing infection, especially by HIV.

Microorganism: a living being of such small size that it can't be seen with the naked eye and is only visible through a microscope, for example viruses and bacteria.

MRSA: *Staphylococcus aureus* that is resistant to methicillin, and the most common among bacteria that are resistant to several antibiotics.

Neuraminidase: a protein of the influenza virus capsule that allows the virus to be released from its host cell to go and infect others. There are nine types and it is one of the antigens used to make vaccines. There are antivirals that inhibit its function. It is abbreviated as N.

Outbreak: a localized infection among a small group of people, like a family, a school or even a village.

Pandemic: an epidemic that has spread across a whole continent, or even the entire planet.

Plasmids: isolated genes of the microbe's genome that can be exchanged with other microorganisms.

Reservoir: a place where microbes can accumulate and from which they can infect humans again in future. Very often the animals that act as reservoirs aren't affected by the presence of the microbe, so show no symptoms of disease.

Resistance: a mechanism by means of which a bacterium ceases to be susceptible to the drug that normally kills or inhibits it.

R0: the sum of new contagions each infected person can cause on average. In other words, the number of people that can catch the microbial infection from each individual who already has it.

Seasonal flu: an annual influenza outbreak that starts with the onset of cold weather and ends around springtime.

Seropositive: a person who has been infected by a microbe and has antibodies against it in the bloodstream. Frequently used to refer to HIV-positive people.

Strain: variant of a microorganism of particular genetic characteristics; for example, a strain of the influenza virus.

Virulence: aggressiveness of a microbe, defined by the gravity of the symptoms it causes.

XDR (extensively drug-resistant): designating a type of MDR that is resistant to most of the commonly used antibiotics.

Index